REALISTIC
BARIATRIC NUTRITION

Realistic
BARIATRIC NUTRITION:
HEALTHY RECIPES AND NUTRITION GUIDELINES AFTER GASTRIC BYPASS AND SLEEVE GASTRECTOMY SURGERY

Copyright © 2021 by Laurie McBride

All rights reserved.
No part of this book may be reproduced, distributed, or transmitted in any form or by any means, including photocopying, recording, or other electronic or mechanical methods, without the prior written permission of the copyright owner except for the use of quotations in a book review.

ISBN: 978-0-578-30787-9

Food photography by: Laurie McBride
Cover Photo by: Amanda Buschman

Disclaimer:
The content of this book is not meant to replace nutrition or medical advice provided by your doctor or medical team. It is recommended that you always keep your doctor informed of what diet you are following and what supplements you are taking and follow any instructions they provide.

To the providers and patients at Northwest Bariatrics who have always encouraged and inspired me to go beyond what I thought I was capable of.

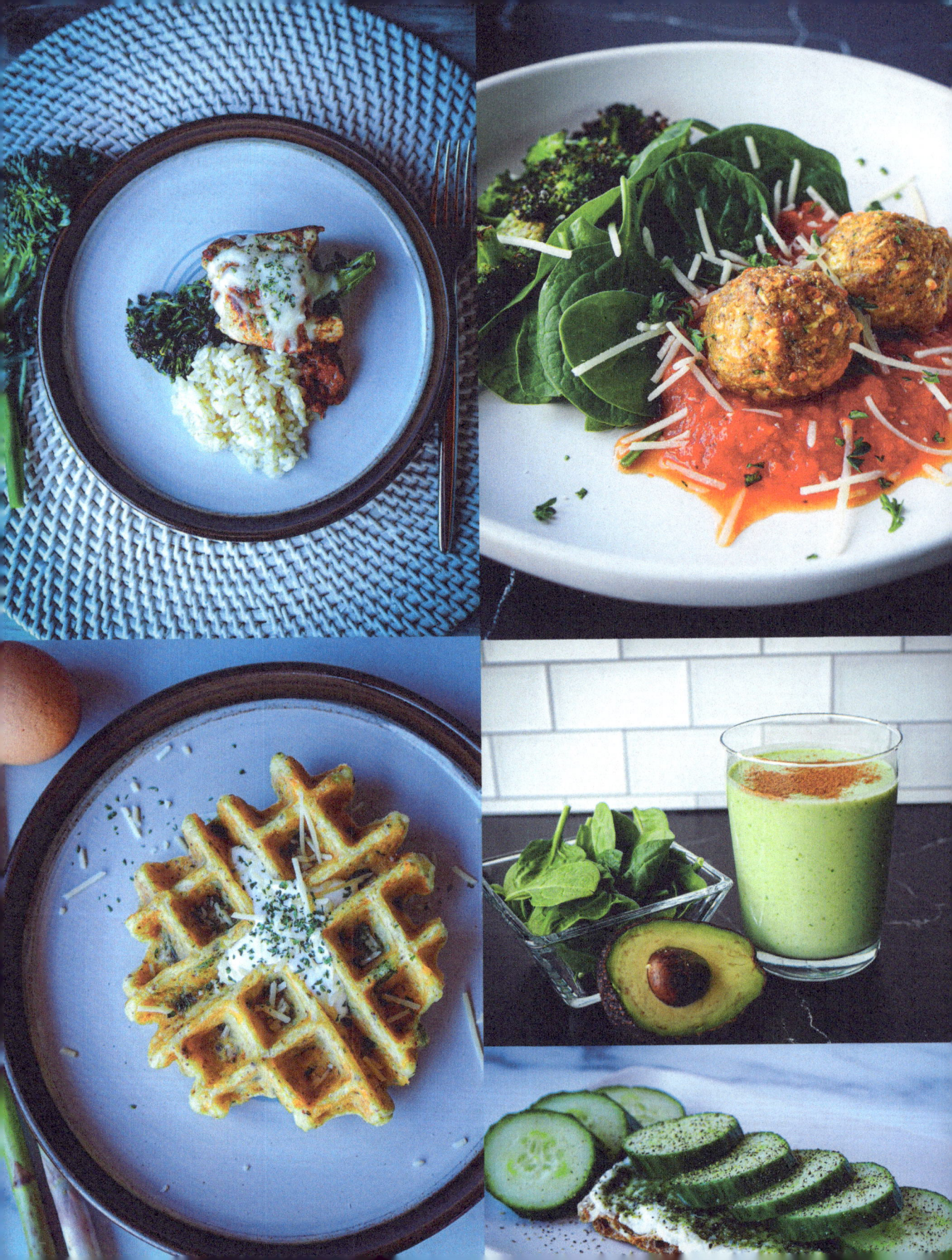

contents

INTRODUCTION
7

PROTEIN SHAKES
31

LIQUID SOUPS
39

PUREED FOODS
49

FRUIT SMOOTHIES
59

BREAKFAST
63

LUNCH
81

DINNER
111

SNACKS
149

MEAL PLANS
157

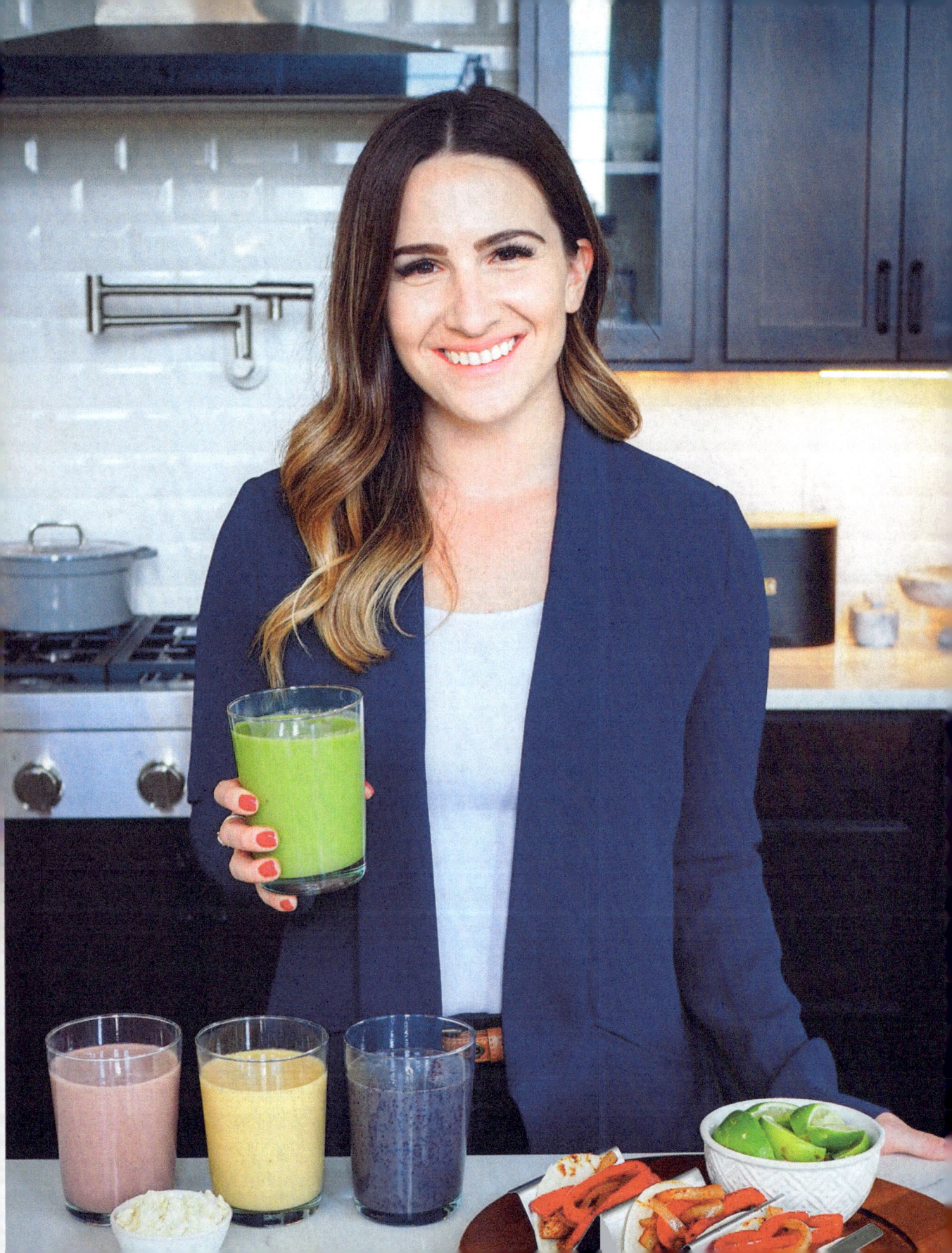

INTRODUCTION

Hello and welcome to Realistic Bariatric Nutrition! I hope this cookbook can be a helpful tool for you to utilize as you start this life-changing experience and pursue weight loss surgery. My name is Laurie. I am a registered dietitian (RD) and have been working in the field of bariatrics for many years. In addition to holding the credential of RD, I am also a certified specialist in obesity and weight management (CSOWM). Prior to my experience in bariatrics, I worked with adults, children, and adolescents on weight management and lifestyle changes to improve their overall health. I have been in the field of weight management for nearly a decade, and it's a field I am very passionate about. I hope with my combined experience of surgical and non-surgical weight loss, I can provide some helpful information and education to prepare you for the changes in your future as you learn to navigate life after bariatric surgery.

Life after surgery can be an overwhelming and exciting process. Some individuals describe it as completely starting over with a clean slate. You have the opportunity to develop new habits and a new lifestyle that supports your health and well-being. You should feel very confident in your decision to pursue weight loss surgery and forget any stigma associated with it. Whenever someone says to me, "I never pursued bariatric surgery because I thought of it as the easy way out," I always challenge those thoughts by pointing out that life after surgery isn't easy, it's hard work. It not only can be difficult physically but it can also be difficult emotionally and psychologically. Have confidence in this decision and know that choosing to pursue surgery is a commitment that will be difficult but worth it.

This book is meant to provide additional guidance for your diet after surgery, tips to consider for long-term weight loss success and simple yet delicious and healthy recipes that are appropriate after bariatric surgery. It is not meant to replace nutritional guidance provided by your surgeon, bariatric team, or bariatric dietitian. Every individual will have different nutritional needs based on their past medical history, weight status, gender, age, etc. If you ever feel like you need additional support regarding your diet or have concerns about your surgery, I strongly encourage you to follow up with your bariatric surgery clinic and dietitian. This book is simply to supplement the guidance and education that has been provided to you by your bariatric team.

Introduction
NUTRITION PHILOSOPHY

I thought I would start by introducing to you my philosophy about nutrition and weight loss. You will notice throughout my book various recipes that include high-carbohydrate foods like beans, fruit (yes, even bananas), potatoes, and other "forbidden" foods the weight loss industry tells us to avoid. Realistic bariatric nutrition is meant to be just that, realistic. Realistic to apply to your life and realistic to maintain throughout your life. I am not a registered dietitian who fears food groups or encourages eliminating entire macronutrients (i.e. carbohydrates). All foods fit within a healthy diet, even after bariatric surgery. You may see a shift of focusing on higher protein foods and trying to limit fat and simple carbohydrates after surgery, usually because these foods are not well tolerated. But it's a good idea to remind yourself that every person's experience, food preferences, and food intolerances are very different after surgery. It is always my goal to guide each patient toward a general healthy diet that is realistic for them to maintain after weight loss surgery, as the chronic dieting and unrealistic food rules are now a thing of the past.

Food is meant to be fuel for our body, but food is also meant to be enjoyed. Many of my patients have tried diets consisting of foods they genuinely dislike. How is someone going to stick to a diet they hate and doesn't taste good to them? Willpower? You may have heard this before, but experts consider willpower a muscle, because it does fatigue. Therefore, having a goal to rely on your willpower alone to choose healthy foods isn't a very realistic goal. Creating an environment that makes healthy eating an easy decision is the ultimate goal. A healthy diet needs to be easy to follow, and it needs to be enjoyable. If it's not easy to follow and if you don't enjoy the foods you're eating, you most likely won't follow it for long.

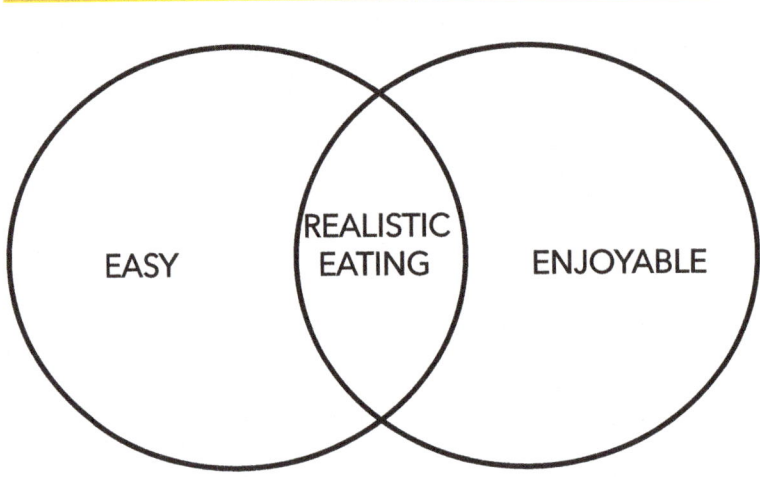

BARIATRIC SURGERY: A TOOL FOR WEIGHT LOSS

I have been in the weight management world since I became a dietitian. I have been exposed to thousands of patients and their stories of struggling with their weight, constantly following the latest fad diet and being on this up and down roller coaster of losing and gaining the same amount of weight for decades. It can be exhausting and very discouraging, which is why, more and more individuals are turning toward bariatric surgery as a long-term solution for weight management. But it's important to realize that bariatric surgery is not a magic pill and your bariatric surgeon isn't going to wave their wand and give you the results you are wanting. Realistic lifestyle changes that are sustainable to maintain lifelong are going to give you the results you want in the short-term and long-term. These lifestyle changes aren't easy. Changing behaviors and changing habits is very difficult, which is why, I believe working with a mental health expert can be very beneficial during this process. But there are tools that can help you achieve healthier lifestyle patterns and help with your weight loss journey, and you should think of bariatric surgery as one of these tools. You will utilize this tool along with other tools to help you achieve your weight loss goal and long-term weight maintenance.

During this first section we will discuss weight management strategies, tools to help you achieve your weight loss goal and various nutrition concepts especially related to bariatric surgery. Let's first discuss a little more of how bariatric surgery works to help you understand how your body will be changing.

BARIATRIC SURGERY: HOW IT WORKS

Weight loss surgery helps individuals follow a low calorie diet to promote weight loss and a balanced calorie diet to promote weight maintenance. The main mechanism of how surgery helps with weight loss is hormonal shifts in the gastrointestinal tract. An individual with normal anatomy who does not get bariatric surgery may struggle with following a low calorie diet for a period of time. The reason why this can be difficult is because our body hates losing weight and tries to prevent it as much as possible. When creating a calorie deficit, your body will start increasing production of the appetite stimulating hormone, ghrelin, to increase calorie consumption and stop weight loss.[2] With bariatric surgery, this mechanism is reversed and, the body will not produce as much appetite stimulating hormone, thus decreasing appetite.[3] Most individuals after surgery will report having a minimal appetite, especially immediately after surgery. In addition to this change in ghrelin production, bariatric surgery causes food to move more quickly through the gastrointestinal tract. The rapid introduction of food into the small intestine will increase production of hormones that produce feelings of fullness.[4] Therefore, after surgery, most individuals would have a limited appetite and get very full, very quickly. However the benefit of these hormone changes may not be permanent. This is why focusing on your weight loss efforts during the initial twelve to eighteen months after surgery is important. These hormone changes in the gastrointestinal tract is the main mechanism of how bariatric surgery works to help individuals achieve substantial weight loss.

HORMONE CHANGES AFTER BARIATRIC SURGERY:

↑ FEELINGS OF FULLNESS   ↓ APPETITE AND HUNGER

NUTRITION 101

In order to understand what your diet will look after surgery, you will need to understand some basic nutrition concepts. Keep in mind, everyone's nutritional needs will be slightly different. The information provided below is an example of calorie/macronutrient distribution for most individuals after weight loss surgery, not all individuals. Please seek additional guidance from your dietitian.

We have all heard and know the term "calories." But do you know what calories actually are? No, they are not little gremlins that come out at night and sew your clothes tighter and tighter. A calorie is a unit of energy, therefore you will hear the term *calorie* and the term *energy* interchangeably. We all need a specific amount of calories in order to support basic functions like breathing, digesting food, walking, thinking, etc. So no, you should not go to the gym and burn 1200 calories because you ate 1200 calories. If you did this, your body would have no energy to perform basic functions. It is when we consume too many calories that our body begins to gain weight unintentionally and creating a calorie deficit is needed to help you lose weight. Everyone's calorie needs are very different, and I encourage you to reach out to your dietitian if you are interested in knowing your specific caloric needs.

There are three macronutrients that provide calories, and I bet you have heard of all three: protein, carbohydrates and fat. So whenever you are consuming calories, you need to think about how those calories are coming from either protein, carbohydrates, or fat in your food. Knowing this concept will help you with planning meals and balancing your macronutrients.
Protein provides 4 calories per 1 gram. For example, a protein shake that contains 30g of protein will contain 120 calories from protein. After bariatric surgery, I usually rec-

ommend 30% of your calories come from protein for most individuals.

Carbohydrates provide 4 calories per 1 gram. For example, that same protein shake that contains 5g of carbohydrates will contain 20 calories from carbohydrates. After bariatric surgery, I usually recommend that 40% of calories come from carbohydrates for most individuals. Yes! You want slightly more calories coming from carbohydrates, which may be a surprise for most people who have chronically dieted throughout their life. This macronutrient is the body's main energy source, among other health benefits, so having healthy carbohydrates in your diet is important.

Fat provides 9 calories per 1 gram. Let's take the same example as before, and this protein shake also contains 5g of fat, therefore it contains 45 calories from fat.

Macronutrient Distribution Recommendation after Surgery:

PROTEIN	CARBOHYDRATES	FAT
30% OF CALORIES	40% OF CALORIES	30% OF CALORIES

Based on a 1200 calorie per day diet, this would be 90g protein (360 calories from protein), 120g carbohydrates (480 calories from carbohydrates), and 40g fat (360 calories from fat). Keep in mind these macronutrient distributions are applicable long-term after surgery and not immediately after surgery when your diet is very limited and high in protein. It's typical immediately after surgery to have a diet that is 50-60% protein to ensure protein needs are being met while consuming a very low calorie diet.

You don't have to count macronutrients ("macros"). This information is only being provided if you are curious to know how they can be distributed after surgery. Utilizing some form of self-monitoring with your diet is highly recommended after surgery however there are many ways you can do this, which we will review in a later section.

EATING AFTER SURGERY

POST-SURGICAL PROGRESSION DIET
After surgery, you will go through what I like to call a post-surgical progression diet for the first one to two months. This usually means going from liquids, to pureed foods, to soft foods and eventually to a general diet as tolerated. This progression diet varies between every bariatric program therefore I will not provide information of how to progress your diet after surgery. Please follow your surgeon's protocol at your bariatric surgery clinic.

PORTION SIZES

After surgery, you will be very limited in portion sizes, not only of solid foods but with liquids as well. There will be a time after surgery when you can only consume about 1/4 cup of total food per meal, and individuals will eventually get to a point when they are able to consume about 1 cup of total food per meal. Patients slowly increase portion sizes as they progress after surgery due to the body adjusting to the new anatomy and adjusting to the hormone shifts in the gastrointestinal tract as previously mentioned, and portion sizes are going to be very individualized.

Usually two to four months after surgery, I see patients being able to tolerate about 1/2-3/4 cup total food per meal. This will increase to 1 cup total food per meal anytime between four to seven months after surgery, sometimes longer. Make sure to read your internal fullness cues and not get overly full after meals. This should be driving your portion sizes. If you are feeling satisfied after 1/2 cup of food, then this will be an appropriate portion size for you. You may also find the type of food you are eating will drive your portion sizes. Patients will get full more quickly and with less food when they are eating a high-protein, high-fiber meal. If patients are eating a meal lower in protein and/or fiber, they may be able to eat more of it.

MEAL FREQUENCY

Within the first few months after surgery when your portion sizes are the smallest, you may need to have about five small meals/snacks during the day. Once portion sizes get to 1/2-1 cup total food per meal I usually recommend four to five small meals/snacks during the day with no grazing behaviors in between. It's important to establish structure with your meals and limit mindless eating and snacking throughout the day. I usually recommend spreading out your meals/snacks over a ten to twelve hour window with your first meal starting within one to two hours of waking up. Here is an example of how to schedule your meals after surgery:

7am	Wake up
8am	Meal #1
10am	Snack #1
12pm	Meal #2
3pm	Snack #2 (optional)
6pm	Meal #3
10pm	Sleep

**For examples of meals after surgery please refer to the meal plans section on page 157

EATING BEHAVIORS AFTER SURGERY

Like previously mentioned, food intake after surgery needs to be structured and well planned. Mindless snacking and grazing needs to be limited, as these behaviors can cause issues with tracking intake and overall weight management. They can also be problematic in regards to uncomfortable gastrointestinal symptoms. Make sure your food intake is intentional, mindful, and structured.

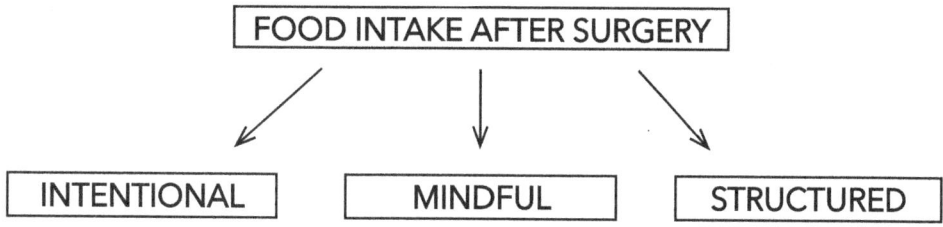

One behavior to begin practicing before surgery is slowing down during mealtimes. It's so easy to go into autopilot while eating when maybe you are eating too quickly or taking too large of bites. This can cause gastrointestinal symptoms after surgery and also lead to feelings of being too full and sometimes even feeling sick after meals. Begin practicing taking small bites, chewing foods very well before swallowing and eating foods slowly. I usually recommend patients take about 30 minutes to eat a meal after surgery. However, you don't want to take too long to eat your meals. When patients are taking 45 minutes or longer to eat a meal, they are able to eat larger portion sizes because food begins to move through the gastrointestinal tract, therefore making room for more food. Try to go into each meal with a plan of what your meal will consist of, measure out your portions, give yourself time to eat your meal (around 30 minutes), stop when you are satisfied, and then step away from the meal. All of this may seem overwhelming initially, but once you practice this over the course of several months, it will become a new habit.

DRINKING FLUIDS

A common struggle for most patients after surgery is drinking adequate fluids. Fluid intake and maintaining adequate hydration should be every bariatric patient's number one priority because one of the most common reasons for hospital readmission after surgery is dehydration.[1] The reason fluid intake can be difficult is because patients are unable to gulp or guzzle fluids and liquids can be very filling after surgery. Due to the new anatomy, patients need to take small sips of fluids all day long, therefore you need to start the habit of carrying water with you wherever you go. Preferred fluids after surgery to promote adequate hydration is any calorie-free clear liquid like water or sugar-free sports drinks. Patients may also include sugar-free additives to their water if they prefer. Protein shakes and other fluids that contain calories should not be counted toward total fluid intake. I usually recommend patients get a minimum of 50 ounces[7] after surgery; however, I recommend aiming for at least 64 ounces after surgery to ensure adequate hydration. It is possible to drink more fluids. Some patients feel better when drinking 80 or more ounces during the day but this will be individualized. When visiting with your bariatric dietitian ask how much fluid they recommend after surgery and what an appropriate goal should be for you.

In addition to only being able to drink small sips throughout the day, patients should separate food and fluid intake. There are two reasons why separating food and fluids is important. One reason is because drinking fluids while eating can flush food through the gastrointestinal tract too quickly. When this happens it can cause gastrointestinal upset or cause patients to get hungry more quickly after a meal. The second reason to separate food and fluids is to ensure adequate protein, calorie, and nutrient intake. During mealtimes is your time to eat nutrient dense and high-protein foods to meet nutritional needs. You do not want to fill up your stomach with calorie-free liquids during this time. The recommendation I provide patients is not to drink fluids for 15 minutes before they eat or for 30 minutes after they eat. If you are eating approximately four meals daily, this causes four separate time frames when you are unable to drink any fluids to aid in hydration. Pair this with only being able to drink small sips at a time, and you will begin to understand why fluid intake can be very challenging after bariatric surgery.

> **NUMBER ONE NUTRITION PRIORITY= WATER/CALORIE-FREE LIQUIDS**
>
> **GOAL= 64 OUNCES DAILY**

FOOD INTOLERANCES

Food intolerances after surgery can be frustrating and difficult to manage. Some individuals after surgery can eat anything and everything without any issues, and some individuals struggle with what seems like anything they consume. I define a food intolerance as any food that causes gastrointestinal upset after it is consumed (vomiting, nausea, diarrhea, regurgitation, bloating, discomfort). Although many of these symptoms can be a normal part of adjusting to life after surgery, they can also be indicative of a complication. I recommend communicating any concerns to your bariatric program. However, if you feel like some foods just aren't "agreeing" with your new anatomy, this can be very normal after surgery but still an unpleasant thing to manage. I mostly observe food intolerances during the initial few months after surgery and these intolerances can resolve on their own with time. Although less often, these food intolerances have the potential to be long-term.

What causes food intolerances after surgery? It could be your gastrointestinal tract healing or getting familiar with the new anatomy, but it also could be the way you are eating food. Like previously mentioned, it can be easy to go into autopilot or get distracted while eating, causing you to take too large of bites, not chewing foods enough, or eating foods too quickly. Check in with yourself and evaluate whether these eating patterns could be the reason for any intolerances you are experiencing and make sure to be very mindful during all eating occurrences. Also, ensure you are advancing your diet per your bariatric surgery program. It is very important to not advance your diet too quickly.

One specific intolerance I see most is an intolerance to dairy. Bariatric surgery can worsen lactose intolerance symptoms, and I've also seen it cause new incidences of lactose intolerance. The degree of lactose intolerance can vary. Some people tolerate cheese or yogurt but are unable to tolerate milk while others need to cut dairy out of their diet completely. If you struggle with lactose intolerance before surgery, be mindful of how your body responds when reintroducing it after surgery.

The bottom line when it comes to food intolerances is they are very individualized and difficult to predict. When advancing your diet after surgery, try new foods slowly and in small amounts. In addition to this, make sure you are taking small bites, chewing foods well, and being mindful during meals by avoiding distractions. Follow up with your bariatric surgery clinic to better define whether you are experiencing food intolerances or a possible surgical complication. And another piece of advice, don't try a new food while out and about, just in case things don't go as planned and you need a bathroom quickly.

PROTEIN SHAKES AND SUPPLEMENTS

If you are not already familiar with protein shakes and supplements, it will be a good idea for you to begin familiarizing yourself with these products. Protein supplements are a significant part of the pre-surgical and post-surgical diet, and making sure you are meeting your protein needs after surgery will be an important priority (aside from staying hydrated, of course). When deciding which protein supplements to use, you want to think about the purpose your protein supplement will be serving in your diet. Are you using protein shakes as meal replacements on a liquid diet? Are you using a protein supplement to supplement or boost your protein intake? Let's discuss the different types of protein supplements and how or whether to include them in your diet after surgery.

Protein Shakes

This will probably be the most common protein supplement you will use after surgery. Protein shakes come in cartons/bottles that are already in liquid form. You just crack them open and enjoy. They also come in powder form and you have to do the mixing yourself. Usually patients are using protein shakes as meal replacements so there are guidelines you want to consider when using them as meals:

Protein shakes as meal replacements:

200 calories	20-30g protein	Variety of vitamins and minerals

Meal replacement shakes are easily available; you can find them at virtually any grocery store and also online. You should plan on utilizing these while on liquid diets, but you can also utilize them as a convenient meal replacement in the long-term. It's always my recommendation to keep your doctor and bariatric dietitian informed of what supplements you are utilizing as meal replacements to ensure nutritional adequacy and follow any recommendations they provide.

Protein Waters
These supplements are increasing in popularity and are being used by bariatric patients more often. Protein waters can be a helpful boost when you are having trouble meeting your protein needs; however, there are some considerations you want to keep in mind.

Protein water is not a significant source of vitamins and minerals and does not contain essential nutrients. Therefore, these products should not be used as meal replacements. With that said, usually these products are being consumed in addition to normal meals and snacks, which can contribute to additional calories during the day (as opposed to drinking calorie-free options). Sometimes, these added calories and protein can be beneficial (for example early post-surgery when it's difficult to consume enough calories and protein), but in the long run, to ensure success with weight maintenance, you want to prevent excess calorie consumption which can lead to weight regain.

If you are utilizing these supplements for a boost in protein intake, make sure you are getting a high-quality protein. Most protein waters on the shelf today are being made with whey protein isolate, which is a high-quality protein. However in the past there have been protein waters that are made with collagen. Avoid these protein waters because collagen is not a complete protein. Therefore, you will not be consuming all essential amino acids, and these incomplete proteins should not be counted toward your total protein intake.

Another consideration is added sugar. Most protein waters that I have seen do include small amounts of added sugar. Usually not quite in the amount of soda or fruit juice but nonetheless, added sugar. The bottom line is, you may use protein water if you need to boost protein intake but if you are meeting protein needs with your meals/snacks, then you are probably better off choosing a calorie-free option.

Protein Powders
There are many options available if you are looking for a protein powder to utilize. I categorize protein powders as either meal replacement powders or protein supplements/boosters, and when choosing a protein powder, think about how you will be utilizing it.

Meal replacement powders should follow the same guidelines as meal replacement shakes in the previous section. I usually recommend these powders if you are on a liquid diet and will only be mixing these powders with water or something like unsweetened almond milk. I don't recommend these powders when using them as a protein source in things like fruit smoothies. If you are looking for a protein supplement to utilize in a smoothie, try getting a protein powder that is 100 calories or less and 20-30g of protein. These powders will serve as your protein source and pairs well with your other additives like fruit, milk, or yogurt.

It is also worth mentioning in this section that protein shakes, protein powders, and protein waters all have whey-based options and plant-based options. If you are unable to tolerate whey-based protein supplements then try a plant-based protein supplement and work with your dietitian to figure out something that works for you.

Protein Bars
Are they protein bars or glorified candy bars? These protein supplements are not ones that I recommend often to patients. When looking at the nutrition label of a protein bar, you may find a lot of resemblance to the candy bars that are for sale right next to them. Usually these products are high in carbohydrates, sugar, and calories. For comparison, I have included the macronutrient composition of a popular protein bar and popular candy bar:

Protein Bar	Candy Bar
Serving size 1 bar	Serving size 1 package
300 calories	210 calories
Total fat 11g	Total fat 12g
Total carbohydrate 29g	Total carbohydrate 24g
Total sugars 16g	Total sugars 22g
Protein 20g	Protein 5g

Does this information surprise you? I recommend trying to utilize whole foods as meals and snacks as much as possible. Protein bars can be a way to meet your protein needs; however, I recommend not forming a habit to utilize them regularly. Whenever you do need to utilize a protein bar for a convenient meal or snack, I recommend trying to aim for around 200 calories and balancing the protein and carbohydrate content (20g of protein, 20g of carbohydrates).

Protein Needs after Surgery

How much protein should you be consuming after surgery? Like previously mentioned, I usually recommend 30% of your calorie needs come from protein. The general guideline after surgery is for most individuals to aim for 60-80g of protein daily; however, like most nutrition needs, this can be individualized. Follow your bariatric surgery program's recommendations for protein intake. Something else to keep in mind after surgery is that more protein is not necessarily a good thing. After surgery, having a high-protein diet is drilled into the brains of all bariatric surgery patients, so most patients think the more the better when it comes to protein. I encourage you to start considering all macronutrients (protein, carbohydrates, and fat) as important parts of your diet and ensuring the appropriate distribution between all of them is key.

Immediately after surgery when you are very limited on portion sizes and the foods you are able to tolerate, it is absolutely appropriate to have a majority of your calorie intake be from protein. However, the further you move away from your surgery date you will notice the more you will be able to eat during a meal (this is because the benefits of those hormone changes are not permanent after surgery). When gradually increasing portion sizes, it is my advice that you do not fill in with more and more protein. Instead, continue to meet your protein needs, and when you are able to eat 3/4 cup or 1 cup of food at once, fill in with other food groups like vegetables, fruits, beans, maybe even a small amount of whole grains. It is these high-fiber foods that will help you feel full and satisfied after meals when paired with a high-protein food. You can use calorie counting apps or websites like the USDA to determine the protein content of the foods you are eating. Here is a list of high-protein foods that are commonly consumed after surgery[9]:

Protein Content of Foods:

Chicken - 2 ounces	15 grams
Beef - 2 ounces	15 grams
Black beans - 1/2 cup	7 grams
Salmon - 2 ounces	11 grams
Eggs - 1	6 grams
Greek yogurt - 6 ounces	12-15 grams
Almonds - 1 ounce	6 grams
Peanut butter - 2 TBSP	8 grams
String cheese -1	7 grams
Dairy milk - 1 cup	8 grams

DUMPING SYNDROME

A gastric bypass procedure can cause what's called dumping syndrome due to the manipulation of the gastrointestinal tract. This specific procedure bypasses the muscle between the stomach and small intestine called the pyloric sphincter. This muscle regulates how food moves from the stomach into the small intestine, and when this muscle is bypassed, it can cause food to move too quickly into the small intestine. The rapid introduction of food into the small intestine can cause both early dumping syndrome and late dumping.

Early dumping syndrome can happen 10-30 minutes after a meal and can cause symptoms like abdominal cramping, nausea, rapid heart rate, and diarrhea.[4] Dietary management of early dumping syndrome includes having small consistent meals during the day, avoiding large portion sizes, eating foods slowly, separate food and fluid consumption, and limiting simple carbohydrates in the diet (sugary foods, white breads, white pastas, etc.). Some patients can also experience these symptoms when eating foods high in fat.

Late dumping syndrome can happen one to three hours after a meal and is also called "reactive hypoglycemia." The quick introduction of food into the small intestine can cause a rapid release of insulin in the blood stream, which can cause low blood sugar levels a couple of hours after eating.[4] These low blood sugars can be dangerous; therefore, if you are experiencing dizziness, light-headedness, or any of the previously mentioned symptoms during this time frame after eating then you should follow up with your bariatric surgery clinic as soon as possible. Dietary management of late dumping syndrome includes balancing meals with protein, fat, and complex carbohydrates (like whole grains, fruits, vegetables, beans) in order to delay the absorption of carbohydrates in the gastrointestinal tract, which will decrease the amount of insulin released at one time. Treatment can also include medication for those with significant reactive hypoglycemia that is unresponsive to dietary management.

VITAMINS AND MINERALS

Bariatric surgery will increase your risk for vitamin and mineral deficiencies due to the limited diet and alteration of how these nutrients are absorbed in the gastrointestinal tract. Vitamin and mineral deficiencies are a concern for most patients who pursue weight loss surgery, and it should be a concern. These surgeries can alter your needs for vitamins and minerals (also referred to as micronutrients) such as vitamin A, vitamin D, iron, vitamin B12, folate, calcium, zinc, thiamine, and other micronutrients.[6] Individuals who are pursuing weight loss surgery need to commit to the supplementation regimen that is recommended by their surgeon or dietitian. These regimens usually include a bariatric formulated multivitamin, and this is what I recommend for most patients after surgery. There are many brands of bariatric multivitamins out there so have a conversation with your dietitian to determine which once would be best for you. Vitamin and mineral needs will vary based on someone's past medical history and also which procedure they are pursuing, so you always want to follow what your doctor and dietitian are recommending for you.

In addition to committing to the supplementation regimen, patients should also commit to long-term monitoring of micronutrient deficiencies. This usually includes lab tests being done regularly by your bariatric program and/or primary care provider. I always tell my patients the three ways to prevent deficiencies after surgery:

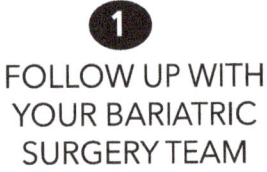
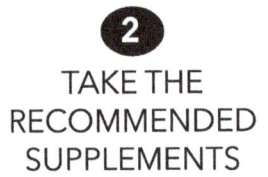
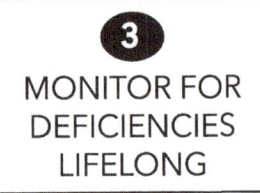

Keep in mind you can follow the supplementation regimen, eat a nutrient dense diet, follow up with your bariatric program as recommended, and still develop a nutrient deficiency someday. This is why it is recommended to monitor vitamin and mineral status lifelong after surgery.

MEAL PLANNING

In my opinion, meal planning is one of the most important parts of weight management, especially after weight loss surgery. I'm sure you have heard the saying, failing to plan is planning to fail. This is something I repeat often to my patients because learning how to plan your meals and snacks will help you maintain a healthy diet throughout your life. Unfortunately we live in an unhealthy society where eating unhealthy is the easy choice. Due to this reality, meal planning is the absolute key to ensure an adequate diet that meets your nutritional needs and supports you in your weight management efforts.

I know meal planning can seem like an inconvenience and never-ending task. Once you have a plan for one week, you have to do it all over again the next week. It's something that can be difficult to get in the habit of, but once you do make it a habit, it won't seem so time-consuming.

Once you are on a general diet after surgery, I recommend including about four to five small meals daily. For every meal, you should aim for a balance of different foods/food groups (rather than only including a protein option). I recommend patients to include at least 2-3 ounces of protein and 1/4-1/2 cup of a fiber source (fruits, vegetables, whole grains).

Developing meal planning skills is very valuable and necessary to experience weight maintenance. You won't be visiting with a dietitian once monthly for the rest of your life therefore you should start developing your own ability to plan meals/snacks. Advice I have for meal planning is to write out your plan each week, think ahead about what events/commitments you have and when you will have time to cook/food prep, and set realistic goals for yourself to follow the meal plan 80% or 90% of the time. Be understanding that life happens, and you won't be able to execute the plan perfectly each week. There are a few strategies for meal planning, you can meal plan one day at a time, a couple of days at a time, or a week in advance. Explore what strategy would be most realistic for you and allow your meal plan to drive your grocery list. For examples of meal plans after surgery please refer to page 157.

SETTING GOALS AND MANAGING EXPECTATIONS

As you begin your journey towards bariatric surgery, it is a good idea to have a conversation with your surgeon about setting realistic goals and expectations after surgery. Patients can enter a bariatric surgery program with a goal of being the weight they were in high school or on their wedding day, and sometimes these goals are unrealistic. When setting weight loss goals, nutrition goals, exercise goals, etc., make sure they are achievable and realistic. Reassessing goals and continuing to have these conversations during your post-surgery follow up appointments can prevent discouragement and feelings of failure.

Consider setting long-term goals and short-term goals. Your long-term goals would include your weight goal and anything else you want to achieve as a result of losing weight. This could include hiking to the top of a mountain, riding a roller coaster with your children, not having to use a seat belt extender on an airplane, being able to cross your legs while sitting, or being able to have your grandchildren sit on your lap. I find these more subjective goals are more motivating than only focusing on the number on the scale alone. I recommend writing down your goals in a journal to help you focus and feel encouraged as you move through the post-surgery phase.

When setting long-term goals consider using the acronym SMART goals. This will ensure your goals are realistic and will also keep your goals focused and specific to clearly define what the goal is and whether or not you have achieved this goal.

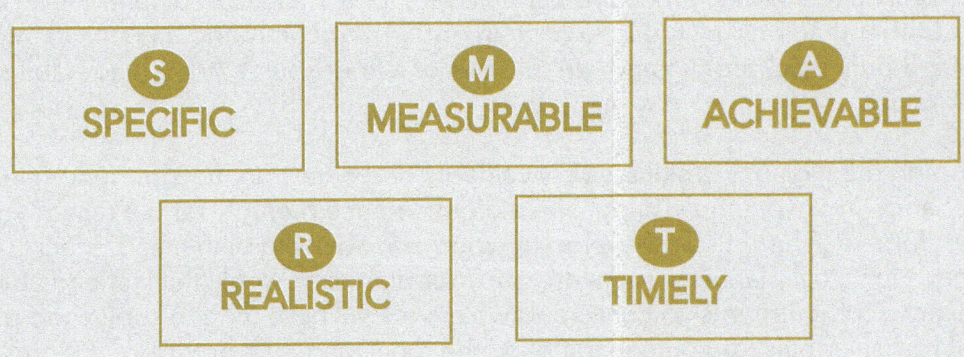

Example of a SMART goal:
I want to hike Mineral Ridge National Recreation Trail and complete the full three-mile loop within two hours by the end of this year.
Example of a SMART goal:
I want to climb ten flights of stairs without stopping for a break within the next three to four months.

In addition to these long-term goals, your short-term goals should be action plans of how you will achieve the long-term goals. Set goals for yourself weekly, monthly, and yearly, and use non-food rewards to celebrate achieving a goal.

Action plan for SMART goal #1:
Begin going on one 30-minute hike per week over the next four weeks. Then increase

this to two 40-minute hikes per week over the following four weeks.
Action plan for SMART goal #2:
Begin taking the stairs at work and only use the elevator one time weekly.

On the topic of goals and expectations, please refrain from comparing yourself to others who have had bariatric surgery. Every patients experience after surgery is very different, and everyone is an individual with their own barriers, goals, past medical history, habits, etc. that you will never know about. This is why setting realistic goals/expectations specific to your situation will be helpful. Another area that can be troublesome in regards to managing expectations is social media. Social media platforms have many resources available where users can take part in online groups and discussions, and there are many weight loss surgery groups. These groups have the potential to be helpful but sometimes they do more harm than good. If you are having concerns about your surgery or your progress after surgery, then have these conversations with the experts at your bariatric surgery clinic. Also, if you are constantly comparing yourself to others on social media then maybe reconsider utilizing this as an avenue for support.

LONG-TERM FOLLOW UP

Following up with your bariatric surgery program is highly recommended. During the first one to two years after surgery, you will follow up more frequently but after this time frame, most programs recommend following up annually. Programs want to follow up with patients once yearly lifelong to ensure you are successful with long-term weight maintenance, address any concerns you may have about your surgical history, monitor for nutrient deficiencies, check in with your diet and lifestyle patterns, and to also communicate with you any new recommendations that have been updated. Bariatric surgery is a field that is constantly progressing, and recommendations are always being updated to ensure evidence-based practice is being utilized. Follow up with your program as recommended to stay up to date on these recommendations.

WEIGHT MANAGEMENT

CHRONIC DIETING
Most patients who pursue weight loss surgery are chronic dieters, meaning they have been on every fad diet out there, losing a significant amount of weight just to regain it back once the fad diet is no longer being followed. There is a statement dietitians have been using for years, and the general population is now catching on. That is, diets do not work. The reason why diets don't work is because usually these diets

involve restricting specific foods or food groups in order to create a calorie deficit and experience weight loss. These restrictive eating patterns are usually not realistic for a majority of people to follow long-term, which is why so many people struggle with weight regain after weight loss.

Keep in mind the reasons why you decided to pursue weight loss surgery. Sometimes patients will get back into the chronic dieting behavior after surgery and want to continue following a very low carbohydrate diet or restrict specific foods or food groups. I always tell patients, do not start anything for weight loss if you don't have the confidence to continue doing it for the rest of your life. Setting unrealistic goals and continuing to have a list of forbidden foods will only further your chronic dieting behavior and probably lead to feelings of failure and discouragement, even after weight loss surgery. Work with your dietitian and counselor/mental health provider to kick the chronic dieting mentality and start establishing a healthy relationship with food. Like I mentioned in my nutrition philosophy, all foods fit within a healthy diet. Your diet and lifestyle should not be so black and white. Learn how to incorporate some grey area, and hopefully weight loss surgery will give you the confidence to do so. I find that practice makes perfect regarding testing specific foods and allowing yourself to include unhealthy foods periodically. Being able to have the confidence and skills to include an unhealthy food then get right back on track is the ultimate goal for long-term success.

EMOTIONAL EATING

As you are evaluating your lifestyle patterns and eating behaviors try and identify if there are reasons you are eating unrelated to your biological hunger. One of the most common eating patterns I encounter with patients is emotional eating habits. Emotional eating is a behavior where someone eats as a response and to cope with a specific emotion. These emotions can include sadness, anger, anxiousness, nervousness, and boredom. To begin evaluating whether you are an emotional eater you have to first assess whether you are feeling biologically hungry or not. If you are not feeling physically hungry, then maybe ask yourself what could be driving you to want to eat in that moment. Did you have a stressful day at work? Did you receive bad news? Did a coworker make you angry? All of these situations can drive a person's desire to eat, but all situations do not necessarily warrant food intake.

There are different levels of emotional eating. I've seen patients who tend to want to snack/graze on food between meals when feeling a little anxious. I've also seen patients who rely on food intake as their main coping mechanism which can involve binging on large amounts of food in one sitting. For those who need to work on not utilizing food when feeling slightly anxious, stressed, or angry, begin to practice other coping mechanisms not involving food. Other coping mechanisms can include:

Listening to music	Drawing/doodling	Playing a game
Going for a walk	Meditating	Doing chores
Phoning a friend	Going for a bike ride	Writing a to-do list
Journaling	Reading a book	Breathing exercises

If you are an emotional eater who uses food as your main coping mechanism and this usually involves eating large amounts of food (sometimes called "binging episodes"), then I highly recommend you begin working with a counselor/mental health provider. These significant emotional eating patterns can be difficult to overcome and may postpone your surgery until you are in remission of these behaviors. Holding off on surgery until the binging episodes have stopped is for your own safety and well-being, so make sure you communicate these behaviors to your surgeon.

SELF-MONITORING

I recommend patients to practice some form of self-monitoring during the weight loss phase and weight maintenance phase after surgery. Self-monitoring strategies can include calorie counting, keeping a food journal, practicing portion control, weighing yourself, meal planning, and practicing mindful eating.

During the weight loss phase (usually the first twelve to eighteen months after surgery), it is beneficial for patients to utilize self-monitoring tools like calorie counting, keeping a food journal, measuring foods, and tracking weight loss. This is to ensure patients are consuming enough calories, enough protein, and that their weight loss goals are being met. There are many calorie counting apps available on smartphones, and they even include a way to track water intake, physical activity patterns, and your weigh-ins. Ask your dietitian what app they recommend if you are wanting to utilize this tool after surgery.

I recommend patients weigh themselves one time weekly. Weighing yourself more frequently (for example, daily) can lead to feelings of discouragement because it's normal to have daily weight fluctuations. Weighing yourself once weekly is frequent enough to capture your weight loss progress and prevent feelings of failure during the week.

Once a patient has met their weight loss goal and our goal moving forward is weight maintenance, it's absolutely realistic to utilize other (not so time-consuming) self-monitoring tools. Utilizing tools like mindful eating, meal planning, regular weigh-ins, and portion control are realistic ways to monitor your food intake and weight maintenance for the long-term. It's always my hope that patients do not have to rely on calorie counting for the rest of their life, but utilizing other tools like regular weigh-ins can give you a quick snapshot of how you are doing in your weight maintenance phase. If you notice your weight creeping up slightly, try not to feel too discouraged or be too hard on yourself. Simply check in to see what could be going on to cause the weight gain and schedule an appointment with your bariatric surgery team for further evaluation.

MINDFUL EATING
Mindful eating is an area of weight management that often gets overlooked. Mindful eating is defined as "paying attention to our food, on purpose, moment by moment, without judgment."[5] So many weight loss programs and diets are based on foods that you should be restricting and eating less often in order to create a calorie deficit. However sometimes increasing mindfulness can be the secret to creating a calorie deficit and experiencing weight loss.

Because food is readily available to us at all times and during all hours, it can lead to eating behaviors that are very mindless. Sometimes, when I ask a patient what they typically eat in a day, they are unable to report this information because sometimes they don't even know what they eat in a day. If you are someone who is constantly eating/snacking/grazing during the day (and maybe you aren't even aware of these behaviors yet), start practicing mindful eating. How do you become more mindful? First by thinking and planning food intake for the day (meal planning). This is another benefit to meal planning that it can nourish a sense of mindful food intake during the day.

Once you have structure in how/when/what you are going to eat during the day, begin asking yourself about internal hunger and fullness cues. Are you feeling biologically hungry? Are you beginning to feel full? Checking with your hunger/fullness cues before you eat, while you are eating, and after you eat will be a helpful behavior to start practicing. Reading internal hunger/fullness cues can seem time-consuming at first, but once you are in the habit of honoring your hunger and fullness then this practice will become easy and automatic.

Utilize the hunger scale to determine your hunger and fullness during the day and during mealtimes:

1	2	3	4	5	6	7	8	9	10
OVERLY HUNGRY/ STARVING				SATISFIED				OVERLY FULL/ STUFFED	

Try to avoid both ends of the hunger scale. You don't want to get too hungry during the day because this usually leads to unhealthy food choices and large portion sizes. You also want to avoid getting overly full because this is a sign you ate too much and did not honor your fullness cues during your meal. I recommend staying within 3-7 on the hunger scale.

There is one phase when I recommend that patients somewhat "override" their internal cues. Within the first twelve months after surgery, it is typical to have a minimal appetite and patients often won't feel hunger cues during the day. This doesn't mean you shouldn't be eating or meeting your nutritional needs and this is especially the time when you want to establish structure with your diet. No matter where you are at in this process, you want to make sure to always honor your internal fullness cues and not get overly full after meals. This is true before surgery, after surgery, ten years after surgery, etc.

FOOD ENVIRONMENT

One aspect of weight management that I encourage patients to explore is their food environment. What I consider your food environment is the environments and relationships at home, work, social gatherings, etc. that impact your food choices and eating patterns. Your food environment directly impacts your lifestyle and food intake. Therefore it can be helpful to explore what changes you can make to your food environment that will help you with sustainable healthy eating.

Examples of factors that impact your food environment are: a spouse or family member who brings unhealthy foods home, coworkers bringing unhealthy snacks to the office, having a candy jar on the kitchen counter in plain sight at all hours, the need to take clients out to lunch frequently for work, or a friend that always suggests hitting up the nearest drive thru for a quick lunch. These relationships and environments are unsupportive of your desire to change lifestyle and eating patterns. The best way to gain more control over your food environment is to have conversations with friends, family, and coworkers of how they can support you in your efforts and not having unhealthy foods readily available at home that will tempt you (especially don't have them in plain sight). Other ideas include suggesting a healthy restaurant to grab lunch, plan an activity with friends or family that does not involve food, and when these foods are around, make a conscious effort to practice mindful eating. Ask yourself what impacts your food choices and your food environment? How can you create an environment at home, school, work, etc that makes living a healthier lifestyle easy and convenient?

ABOUT THIS COOKBOOK

The rest of this book includes 100 recipes you can utilize after bariatric surgery. In addition to each recipe, you will see the nutrition information (calories, protein, carbohydrates, and fat) and what stage of diet you are able to utilize that recipe. You will notice a majority of these recipes are for a general diet. The post-surgery progression diet usually only lasts one to two months, therefore I wanted to include recipes that you can utilize in the long-term after bariatric surgery. These recipes are also appropriate for spouses and families. Have your household browse the recipes and cook what looks good to them.

The portion sizes in these recipes are for bariatric surgery patients. However, portion sizes vary with every individual after surgery so you will want to follow your own internal fullness cues and not consume too large of portions.

Post-surgery Progression Diet Definitions:

GENERAL DIET	No dietary restrictions. You can include raw vegetables, raw fruits, tough meats, etc.
SOFT FOODS DIET	Foods need to be well cooked and soft. No crunchy foods or tough meats.
PUREED DIET	Foods need to be the texture of baby food. Usually involves a blender or food processor to reach appropriate consistency.
LIQUID DIET	Liquids need to be thinned out and free of chunks and seeds, aim for the consistency of milk.

**Follow your bariatric surgery program's post-surgery progression diet and do not advance your diet sooner than instructed.

Congratulations on your decision to pursue weight loss surgery and I wish you well in your endeavors! This process can seem overwhelming, but utilize your support system and resources available at your bariatric surgery clinic. I hope you find the following recipes helpful, delicious, and easy to prepare. I enjoyed creating these recipes, and I hope they stimulate inspiration and reassurance that you can enjoy a healthy diet, especially after weight loss surgery.

REFERENCES

1. Aman MW, Stem M, Schweitzer MA, Magnuson TH, Lidor AO. Early hospital readmission after bariatric surgery. Surgical Endoscopy. 2015;30(6):2231-2238. doi:10.1007/s00464-015-4483-4
2. Cummings DE, Weigle DS, Frayo RS, et al. Plasma ghrelin levels after diet-induced weight loss or gastric bypass surgery. New England Journal of Medicine. 2002;346(21):1623-1630. doi:10.1056/nejmoa012908
3. Dimitriadis GK, Randeva MS, Miras AD. Potential hormone mechanisms of bariatric surgery. Current Obesity Reports. 2017;6(3):253-265. doi:10.1007/s13679-017-0276-5
4. Hui C, Bauza GJ, Dhakal A. Dumping syndrome. StatPearls [Internet]. https://www.ncbi.nlm.nih.gov/books/NBK470542/. Published July 2, 2021. Accessed September 8, 2021.
5. Ionut V, Burch M, Youdim A, Bergman RN. Gastrointestinal hormones and bariatric surgery-induced weight loss. Obesity. 2013;21(6):1093-1103. doi:10.1002/oby.20364
6. Nelson JB. Mindful eating: The art of presence while you eat. Diabetes Spectrum. 2017;30(3):171-174. doi:10.2337/ds17-0015
7. Parrott J, Frank L, Rabena R, Craggs-Dino L, Isom KA, Greiman L. American society for metabolic and bariatric Surgery integrated HEALTH nutritional guidelines for the surgical weight Loss Patient 2016 UPDATE: MICRONUTRIENTS. Surgery for Obesity and Related Diseases. 2017;13(5):727-741. doi:10.1016/j.soard.2016.12.018
8. Sherf Dagan S, Goldenshluger A, Globus I, et al. Nutritional recommendations for adult bariatric surgery patients: Clinical practice. Advances in Nutrition: An International Review Journal. 2017;8(2):382-394. doi:10.3945/an.116.014258
9. U.S. Department of Agriculture, Agricultural Research Service. FoodData Central, 2019. fdc.nal.usda.gov.

Part One: Protein Shakes

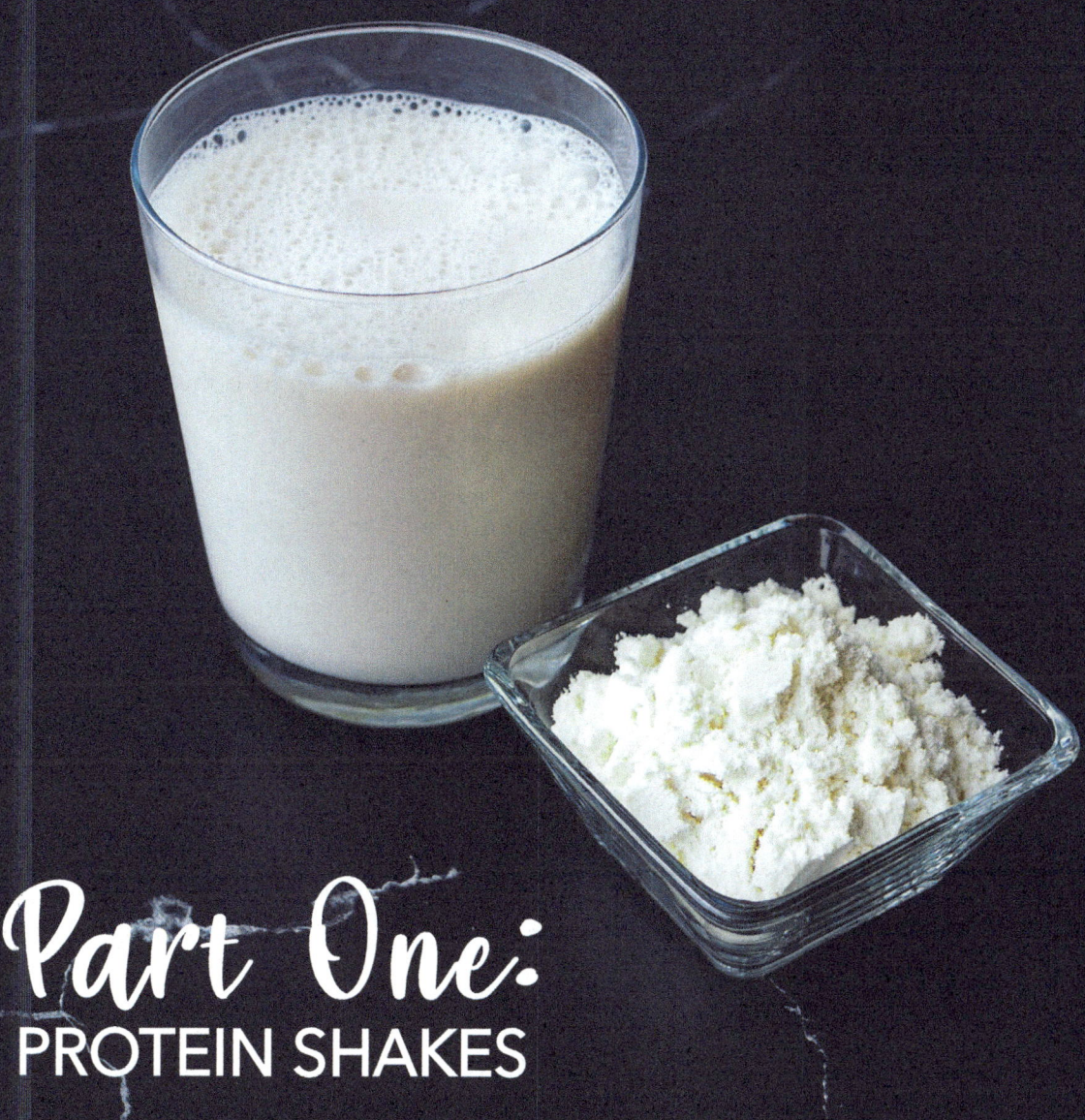

Part One:
PROTEIN SHAKES

Protein powder used in this section meets the following criteria:
2 scoops
150 calories, 30g protein, 2g carbohydrates, 2g fat

Part One: Protein Shakes

ORANGE CREAM

SERVINGS: 1   **MAKES:** 1 PROTEIN SHAKE   **TIME:** 5 MINUTES

INGREDIENTS:

2-4 ice cubes
2 scoops vanilla protein powder
4 ounces low calorie orange juice
4 ounces water
1 TBSP heavy cream

DIRECTIONS:

1. Combine all ingredients in a blender and blend until smooth.

Nutrition Facts:
225 calories, 30g protein, 9g carbohydrates, 7g fat

- LIQUID DIET
- PUREED DIET
- SOFT FOODS DIET
- GENERAL DIET

MOCHA

SERVINGS: 1   **MAKES:** 1 PROTEIN SHAKE   **TIME:** 5 MINUTES

INGREDIENTS:

2-4 ice cubes
2 scoops vanilla protein powder
1 TBSP cocoa powder
1 tsp honey
8 ounces decaf coffee, chilled
1 TBSP heavy cream

DIRECTIONS:

1. Combine all ingredients in a blender and blend until smooth.

Nutrition Facts:
231 calories, 31g protein, 11g carbohydrates, 7.5g fat

- LIQUID DIET
- PUREED DIET
- SOFT FOODS DIET
- GENERAL DIET

Realistic Bariatric Nutrition | 33

LEMON BLUEBERRY

SERVINGS: 1 **MAKES: 1 PROTEIN SHAKE** **TIME: 5 MINUTES**

INGREDIENTS:

2-4 ice cubes
2 scoops vanilla protein powder
1/4 cup fresh or frozen blueberries
1 TBSP lemon juice
1/8 tsp lemon zest
8 ounces cold water

DIRECTIONS:

1. Combine all ingredients in a blender and blend until smooth.

Nutrition Facts:
171 calories, 30g protein, 7g carbohydrates, 2g fat

- LIQUID DIET
- PUREED DIET
- SOFT FOODS DIET
- GENERAL DIET

BANANA NUT

SERVINGS: 1 **MAKES: 1 PROTEIN SHAKE** **TIME: 5 MINUTES**

INGREDIENTS:

1/2 banana
2 scoops vanilla protein powder
4 ounces unsweetened almond milk
4 ounces cold water
1/8 tsp almond extract

DIRECTIONS:

1. Combine all ingredients in a blender and blend until smooth.

Nutrition Facts:
217 calories, 30g protein, 16g carbohydrates, 3g fat

- LIQUID DIET
- PUREED DIET
- SOFT FOODS DIET
- GENERAL DIET

APPLE PIE

SERVINGS: 1 **MAKES:** 1 PROTEIN SHAKE **TIME:** 5 MINUTES

INGREDIENTS:

1 cup oat milk
1 scoop vanilla protein powder
1/4 cup unsweetened applesauce
1/8 tsp cinnamon

DIRECTIONS:

1. Combine all ingredients in a blender and blend until smooth.

Nutrition Facts:
200 calories, 17g protein, 16g carbohydrates, 8g fat

- LIQUID DIET
- PUREED DIET
- SOFT FOODS DIET
- GENERAL DIET

PEACH COBBLER

SERVINGS: 1 **MAKES:** 1 PROTEIN SHAKE **TIME:** 5 MINUTES

INGREDIENTS:

1 cup oat milk
1 scoop vanilla protein powder
1/4 cup peach (frozen or fresh, peeled)
1/8 tsp cinnamon

DIRECTIONS:

1. Combine all ingredients in a blender and blend until smooth.

Nutrition Facts:
190 calories, 17g protein, 13g carbohydrates, 8g fat

- LIQUID DIET
- PUREED DIET
- SOFT FOODS DIET
- GENERAL DIET

COCONUT DREAM

SERVINGS: 1 **MAKES:** 1 PROTEIN SHAKE **TIME:** 5 MINUTES

INGREDIENTS:

1 cup unsweetened coconut milk
2 scoops vanilla protein powder
1 tsp coconut oil

DIRECTIONS:

1. Combine all ingredients in a blender and blend until smooth.

Nutrition Facts:
229 calories, 30g protein, 3g carbohydrates, 10.5g fat

- LIQUID DIET
- PUREED DIET
- SOFT FOODS DIET
- GENERAL DIET

APPLE PEANUT BUTTER

SERVINGS: 1 **MAKES:** 1 PROTEIN SHAKE **TIME:** 5 MINUTES

INGREDIENTS:

1 cup unsweetened almond milk
1/4 cup unsweetened applesauce
1 scoop vanilla protein powder
2 TBSP powdered peanut butter

DIRECTIONS:

1. Combine all ingredients in a blender and blend until smooth.

Nutrition Facts:
200 calories, 24g protein, 13g carbohydrates, 5.5g fat

- LIQUID DIET
- PUREED DIET
- SOFT FOODS DIET
- GENERAL DIET

Part One: Protein Shakes

MINT CHOCOLATE CHIP

SERVINGS: 1   **MAKES:** 1 PROTEIN SHAKE   **TIME:** 5 MINUTES

INGREDIENTS:

1 cup 1% milk
1/4 tsp mint flavor/extract
1.5 TBSP cocoa powder
1 scoop vanilla protein powder

DIRECTIONS:

1. Combine all ingredients in a blender and blend until smooth.

Nutrition Facts:
193 calories, 23g protein, 17g carbohydrates, 3g fat

- LIQUID DIET
- PUREED DIET
- SOFT FOODS DIET
- GENERAL DIET

TROPICAL SUNRISE

SERVINGS: 1   **MAKES:** 1 PROTEIN SHAKE   **TIME:** 5 MINUTES

INGREDIENTS:

4 ounces coconut water
2 ounces pineapple juice
2 ounces low calorie orange juice
2 scoops vanilla protein powder

DIRECTIONS:

1. Combine all ingredients in a blender and blend until smooth.

Nutrition Facts:
222 calories, 30g protein, 19.5g carbohydrates, 2g fat

- LIQUID DIET
- PUREED DIET
- SOFT FOODS DIET
- GENERAL DIET

VANILLA HAZELNUT

SERVINGS: 1 **MAKES:** 1 PROTEIN SHAKE **TIME:** 5 MINUTES

INGREDIENTS:

1 cup 1% milk
1 tsp sugar-free hazelnut syrup
1 scoop vanilla protein powder
1/4 tsp vanilla extract
6 ice cubes

DIRECTIONS:

1. Combine all ingredients in a blender and blend until smooth.

Nutrition Facts:
178 calories, 23g protein, 13g carbohydrates, 3g fat

- LIQUID DIET
- PUREED DIET
- SOFT FOODS DIET
- GENERAL DIET

PUMPKIN CHOCOLATE CHIP

SERVINGS: 1 **MAKES:** 1 PROTEIN SHAKE **TIME:** 10 MINUTES

INGREDIENTS:

2-4 ice cubes
1/4 cup pumpkin puree
2 scoops chocolate protein powder
2 tsp pure maple syrup
1 tsp cocoa powder
1/8 tsp cinnamon
1 cup cold water

DIRECTIONS:

1. Combine all ingredients in a blender and blend until smooth.

Nutrition Facts:
210 calories, 30g protein, 14g carbohydrates, 2g fat

- LIQUID DIET
- PUREED DIET
- SOFT FOODS DIET
- GENERAL DIET

Part Two: Liquid Soups

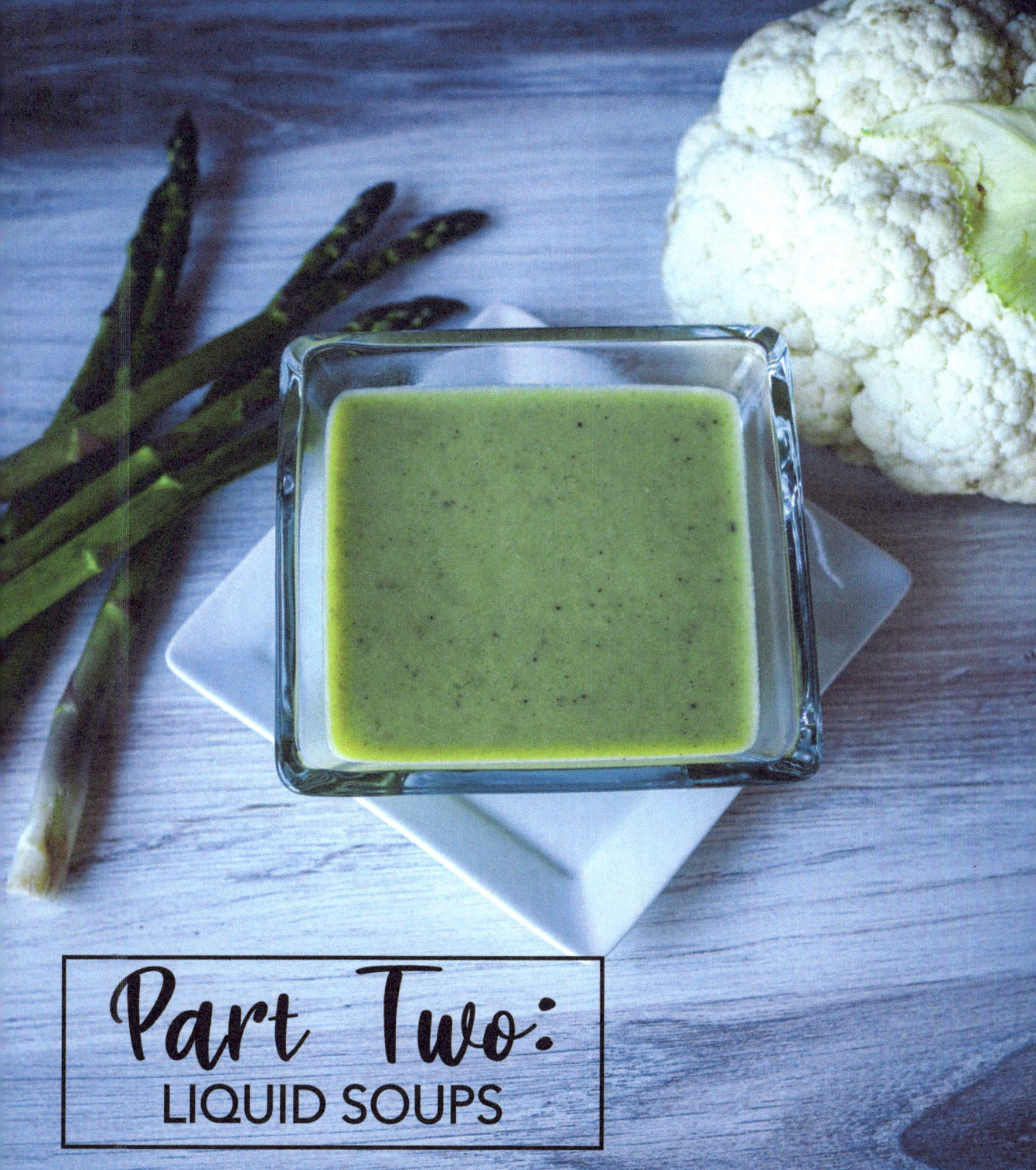

Part Two: LIQUID SOUPS

Unflavored protein powder in this section meets the following criteria:
1 scoop
90 calories, 21g protein

Part Two: Liquid Soups

CAULIFLOWER ASIAGO SOUP

SERVINGS: 6 **MAKES: 3 CUPS** **TIME: 40 MINUTES**

INGREDIENTS:

1 tsp olive oil
1/2 cup onion, chopped
3 cloves garlic, minced
1/2 head cauliflower, chopped
2 cups chicken broth
1/2 tsp salt
1/2 tsp pepper
1/2 tsp Italian seasoning
1/2 cup shredded asiago cheese

Optional Ingredient:
1 scoop unflavored protein powder (per serving)

DIRECTIONS:

1. Heat oil in a large pot over medium-high heat. Once preheated, add the onion and garlic, stir for 2-4 minutes or until the onions begin to look translucent.
2. Add cauliflower to the pot and stir for 1-2 minutes.
3. Add broth, salt, pepper, and Italian seasoning to the pot. Bring to a boil, cover, turn down the heat to low, and simmer for 10 minutes.
4. Uncover the pot and continue to simmer for another 10 minutes.
5. Pierce the cauliflower with a fork to make sure it is soft. When the cauliflower is soft remove pot from the heat and let it cool for 5 minutes.
6. Scoop the contents of the pot into a blender and blend until a smooth consistency.
7. Return the soup to the pot and stir in asiago cheese. Keep stirring until well combined and the cheese is melted.
8. If using protein powder, portion out 1 serving of soup and wait until it is cooled down to less than 140 degrees F. Add 1 scoop protein powder and mix until well combined. My advice is not to include the protein powder until you are ready to eat the soup.

- LIQUID DIET
- PUREED DIET
- SOFT FOODS DIET
- GENERAL DIET

Nutrition Facts (1/2 cup soup + 1 scoop protein powder): 143 calories, 23g protein, 4g carbohydrates, 3g fat

TIPS/SUGGESTIONS:
- You don't have to be on a liquid diet to enjoy this soup! Pair with a small side salad for a yummy lunch even when on a general diet.
- Make ahead of time and portion into mason jars or small containers to enjoy later.

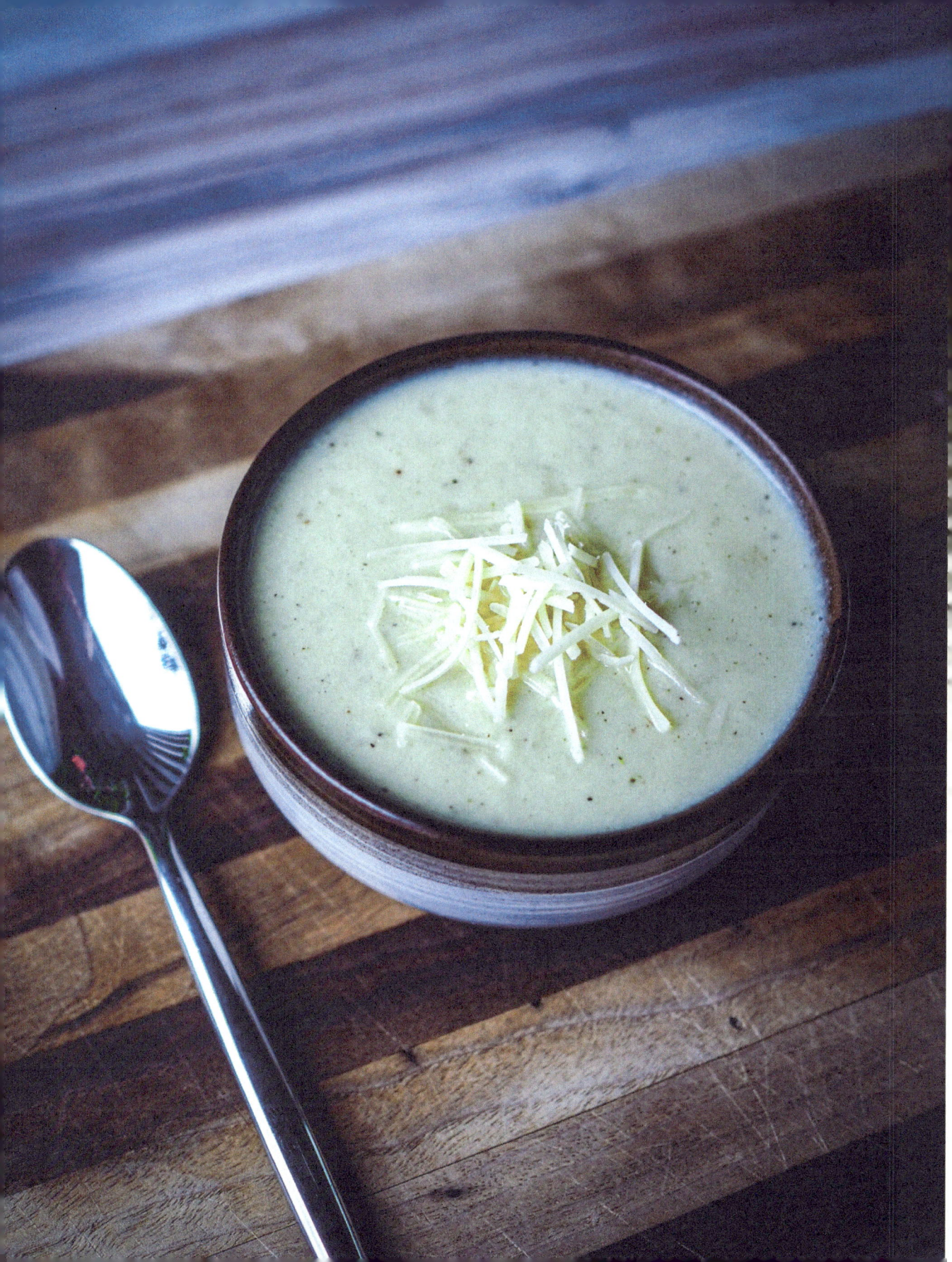

Part Two: Liquid Soups

CARROT GINGER SOUP

SERVINGS: 8 **MAKES: ABOUT 4 CUPS** **TIME: 50 MINUTES**

INGREDIENTS:

1 tsp olive oil
1/2 cup yellow onion, chopped
4 cloves garlic, minced
2 cups carrots, peeled and chopped
1 1/2 cups chicken broth
1/4 tsp salt
1/4 tsp pepper
1/2 tsp ground ginger
1/4 cup unsweetened coconut milk

Optional Ingredient:
1 scoop unflavored protein powder (per serving)

DIRECTIONS:

1. Preheat olive oil in a medium pot over medium heat on the stove top.
2. Add onion and garlic to the pot and cook until fragrant while stirring frequently, about 3-4 minutes.
3. Add the carrots to the pot and cook for another 2-3 minutes, stirring frequently.
4. Pour chicken broth into the pot and bring to a boil. Add salt, pepper, and ground ginger to the soup. Reduce heat and simmer on low for 30 minutes or until carrots are very soft.
5. Remove pot from the heat and let it cool for 5 minutes.
6. Transfer soup to a blender and blend on high until smooth and liquefied.
7. Return mixture to the pot and slowly stir in coconut milk. Portion out about 1/2 cup and let the soup cool down to less than 140 degrees F before stirring in protein powder. Do not add protein powder until ready to eat. Enjoy now or portion out into mason jars or small containers; refrigerate and enjoy later!

- **LIQUID DIET**
- **PUREED DIET**
- **SOFT FOODS DIET**
- **GENERAL DIET**

Nutrition Facts (1/2 cup soup + 1 scoop protein powder): 115 calories, 21g protein, 4g carbohydrates, 1g fat

TIPS/SUGGESTIONS:
- You don't have to be on a liquid diet to enjoy this soup! Pair with a small side salad for a yummy lunch even when on a general diet.

Realistic Bariatric Nutrition | 43

CREAM OF ASPARAGUS SOUP

SERVINGS: 4   **MAKES: 2 CUPS**   **TIME: 40 MINUTES**

INGREDIENTS:

2 tsp olive oil
1 cup asparagus, chopped and ends trimmed
1 cup cauliflower florets, chopped
3 cloves garlic, minced
1/4 tsp salt
1/4 tsp pepper
1/2 tsp dried thyme
1 cup chicken broth
1/4 cup 1% milk

Optional ingredient:
1 scoop unflavored protein powder (per serving)

DIRECTIONS:

1. Preheat olive oil in a medium pot over medium heat on the stove top.
2. Add asparagus, cauliflower, and garlic to the pot. Stir frequently and cook until the vegetables begin to soften, about 3-4 minutes.
3. Add salt, pepper, thyme, and broth to the pot. Bring the mixture to a boil and cover. Reduce heat to low and let the soup simmer for 15 minutes or until the vegetables are soft.
4. Remove the soup from heat and let it cool for 5 minutes. Transfer to a blender or food processor and blend the soup until it's smooth. Return the soup to the pot.
5. Slowly pour in milk while stirring; once the soup is well combined, then you are ready to go.
6. If adding protein powder allow soup to cool down to 140 degrees F before adding protein powder. Do not add protein powder until ready to eat.

- LIQUID DIET
- PUREED DIET
- SOFT FOODS DIET
- GENERAL DIET

Nutrition Facts (1/2 cup soup + 1 scoop protein powder): 134 calories, 23g protein, 4g carbohydrates, 2g fat

TIPS/SUGGESTIONS:
- You don't have to be on a liquid diet to enjoy this soup! Pair with a small side salad for a yummy lunch even when on a general diet.
- Make ahead of time and portion into mason jars or small containers to enjoy later.

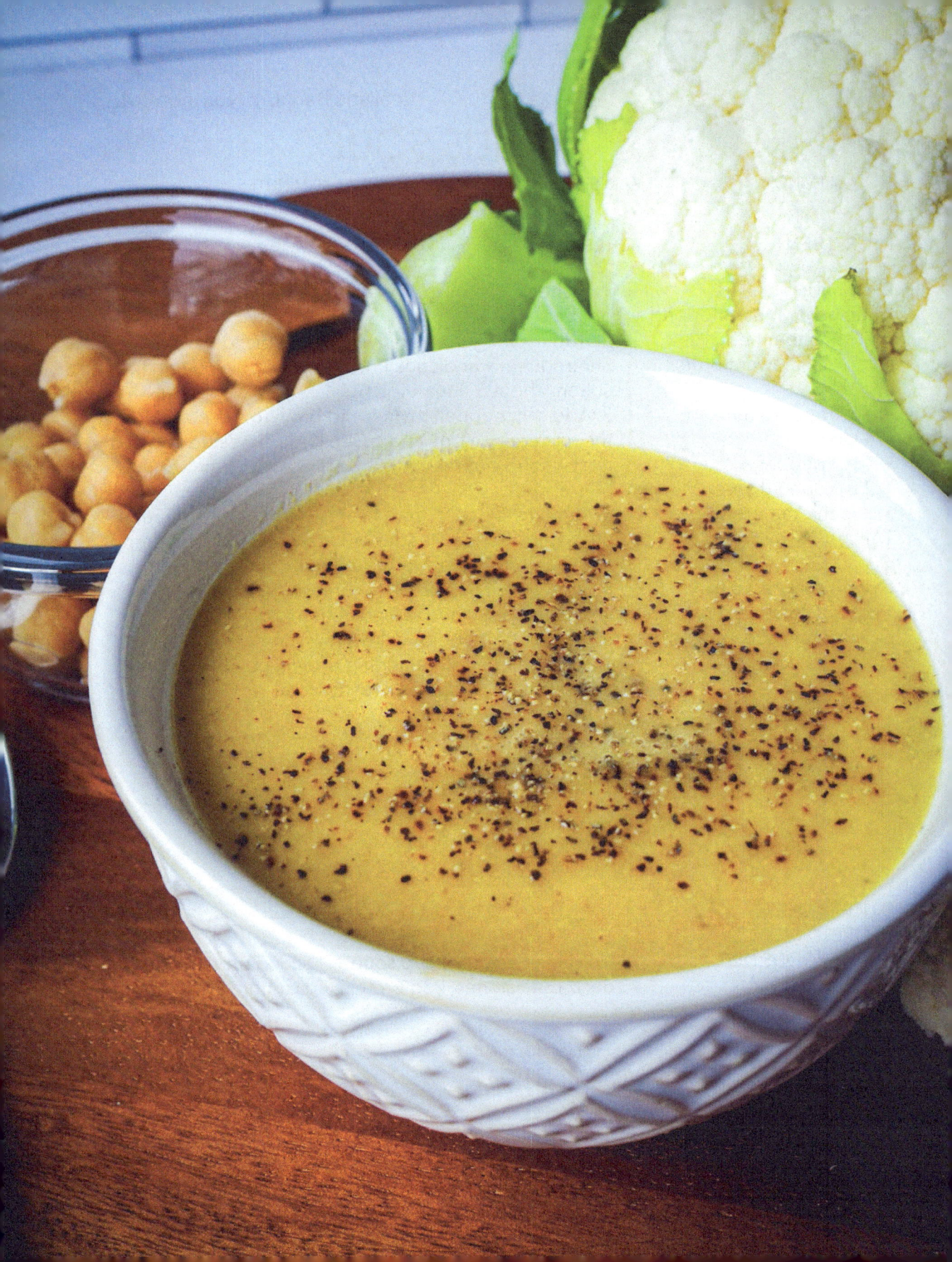

CURRY CHICKPEA SOUP

SERVINGS: 3 **MAKES: 1 1/2 CUPS** **TIME: 40 MINUTES**

INGREDIENTS:

1 tsp olive oil
1/4 cup onion, chopped
1/2 cup cauliflower florets, chopped
1/2 cup canned garbanzo beans, drained and rinsed
1 cup chicken broth
1/8 tsp salt
1/8 tsp pepper
1/2 tsp curry powder
1/8 tsp ginger
1 tsp hot chili sauce

Optional ingredient:
1 scoop unflavored protein powder (per serving)

DIRECTIONS:

1. Preheat a large pot over medium high heat on the stove top and add the olive oil.
2. Add the onion and cauliflower to the pot and stir. Cover the pot and let the vegetables cook for 5 minutes, stirring occasionally.
3. Add garbanzo beans, chicken broth, salt, pepper, curry powder, ginger and hot chili sauce. Bring to a boil, decrease heat to low, and cover. Cook for 15 minutes, stirring occasionally.
4. Remove soup from the heat and allow to cool uncovered for 5 minutes.
5. Transfer mixture to a blender, blend on high until a smooth consistency. Return mixture to the pot, portion out 1/2 cup of the soup and allow to cool to less than 140 degrees F. Mix in 1 scoop protein powder if desired and enjoy. Do not mix in protein powder until ready to eat.

- LIQUID DIET
- PUREED DIET
- SOFT FOODS DIET
- GENERAL DIET

Nutrition Facts (1/2 cup soup + 1 scoop protein powder): 156 calories, 24g protein, 9g carbohydrates, 2.5g fat

TIPS/SUGGESTIONS:
- You don't have to be on a liquid diet to enjoy this soup! Pair with a small side salad for a yummy lunch even when on a general diet.
- Make ahead of time and portion into mason jars or small containers to enjoy later.

Part Two: Liquid Soups

BUTTERNUT SQUASH SOUP

SERVINGS: 4   **MAKES: 2 CUPS**   **TIME: 35 MINUTES**

INGREDIENTS:

2 tsp olive oil
2 cups frozen butternut squash, chopped
1/2 cup onion, chopped
3-4 cloves garlic, minced
1 1/2 cups vegetable broth
1/2 tsp salt
1/4 tsp pepper
1/4 tsp dried sage
1/8 tsp paprika
1/2 tsp dried oregano
1/4 cup lite coconut milk, canned

Optional ingredient:
1 scoop unflavored protein powder (per serving)

DIRECTIONS:

1. In a large pot preheat olive oil over medium-high heat on the stove top.
2. Add butternut squash, onion, and garlic to the pot. Cook while continuously stirring until fragrant and the vegetables begin to soften, about 5-6 minutes.
3. Add broth, salt, pepper, sage, paprika, and oregano to the pot, cover and bring to a boil. Reduce heat to low and simmer for 10 minutes or until the vegetables are soft, stirring occasionally.
4. Remove from heat and allow the soup to cool for about 5 minutes uncovered.
5. Transfer soup to a blender or food processor and blend until a smooth consistency.
6. Transfer soup back to the pot and slowly stir in coconut milk. Season with additional salt/pepper as desired.
7. Portion out 1/2 cup of soup and allow to cool to less than 140 degrees F. Stir in 1 scoop of unflavored protein powder if desired. Do not add in the protein powder until ready to eat.

- LIQUID DIET
- PUREED DIET
- SOFT FOODS DIET
- GENERAL DIET

Nutrition Facts (1/2 cup soup + 1 scoop protein powder): 147 calories, 22g protein, 7.5g carbohydrates, 3g fat

TIPS/SUGGESTIONS:
- You don't have to be on a liquid diet to enjoy this soup! Pair with a small side salad for a yummy lunch even when on a general diet.
- Make ahead of time and portion into mason jars or small containers to enjoy later.

SWEET POTATO BISQUE

SERVINGS: 4 **MAKES: 2 CUPS** **TIME: 35 MINUTES**

INGREDIENTS:

2 tsp olive oil
2 cups sweet potatoes, peeled and chopped
1/2 cup yellow onion, chopped
1 cup vegetable broth
1/4 tsp nutmeg
1/4 tsp dried sage
1/4 tsp dried coriander
1/2 tsp salt
1/4 cup half-and-half milk

Optional ingredient:
1 scoop unflavored protein powder (per serving)

DIRECTIONS:

1. Preheat olive oil in a large pot over medium-high heat on the stove top.
2. Add sweet potatoes and onion to the pot, stir continuously, and cook until the vegetables begin to soften or about 6-8 minutes.
3. Add broth, nutmeg, sage, coriander and salt to the pot. Bring mixture to a boil then reduce heat to low, cover and allow to simmer for 15-20 minutes or until the potatoes are soft and cooked through, stirring occasionally.
4. Remove pot from the heat and allow the soup to cool for about 5 minutes, uncovered.
5. Transfer the mixture to a blender or food processor and blend until a smooth consistency.
6. Return soup to the pot and slowly stir in half-and-half. Season with additional salt as desired.
7. Portion out 1/2 cup of soup and allow to cool to less than 140 degrees F. Stir in 1 scoop of unflavored protein powder if desired. Do not add in the protein powder until ready to eat.

- LIQUID DIET
- PUREED DIET
- SOFT FOODS DIET
- GENERAL DIET

Nutrition Facts (1/2 cup soup + 1 scoop protein powder): 201 calories, 22.5g protein, 17.5g carbohydrates, 4g fat

TIPS/SUGGESTIONS:
- You don't have to be on a liquid diet to enjoy this soup! Pair with a small side salad for a yummy lunch even when on a general diet.
- Make ahead of time and portion into mason jars or small containers to enjoy later.

Part Three: Pureed Foods

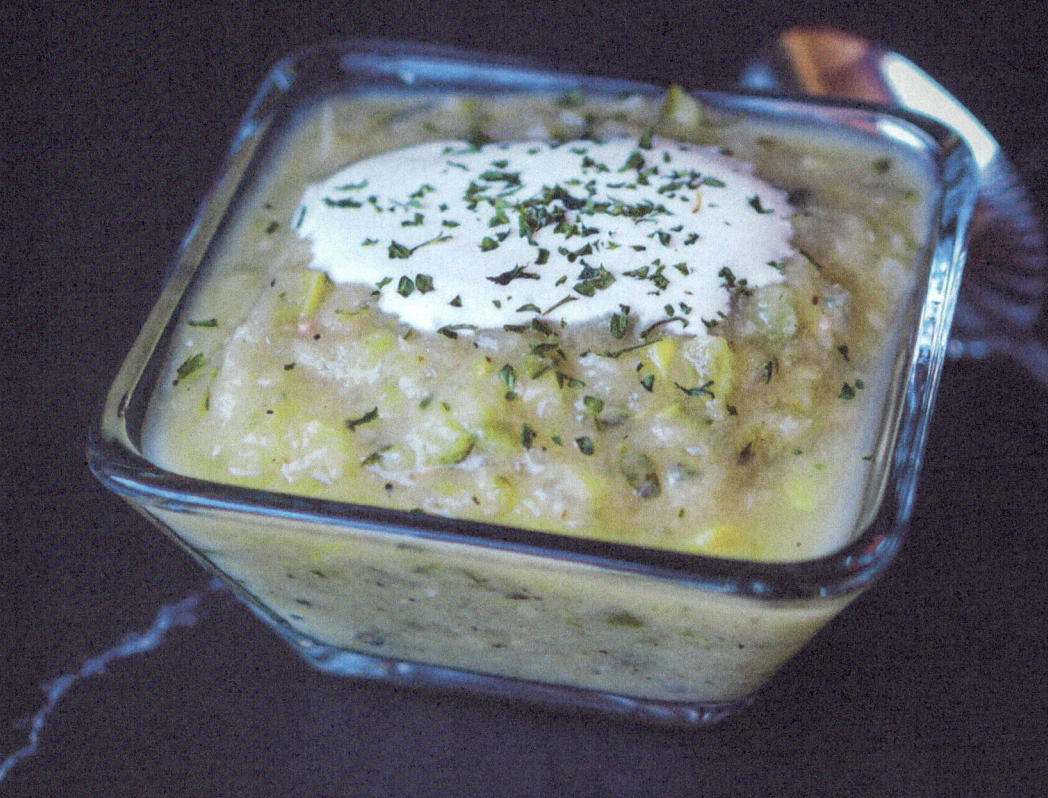

Part Three:
PUREED FOODS

Protein powder used in this section meets the following criteria:
1 scoop
90-100 calories, 20-21g protein

Part Three: Pureed Foods

SOUTHWEST EGGS

SERVINGS: 1 **MAKES: 1/3 CUP** **TIME: 10 MINUTES**

INGREDIENTS:

1 tsp olive oil
1 egg
1 egg white
Pinch of salt and pepper
1/4 tsp garlic
1/4 tsp chili powder
1/8 tsp cumin
1/8 tsp paprika
1 TBSP shredded cheese
2 TBSP fat free refried black beans, warmed

- PUREED DIET
- SOFT FOODS DIET
- GENERAL DIET

DIRECTIONS:

1. Preheat a small pan over medium heat on the stove top and coat with olive oil.
2. In a small bowl, combine egg, egg white, salt, pepper, garlic, chili powder, cumin, and paprika.
3. Whisk together ingredients with a fork until well combined.
4. Pour egg mixture into the pan and stir continuously until the eggs are fluffy and cooked through.
5. Sprinkle cheese over the eggs and serve with refried beans.

Nutrition Facts:
186 calories, 13g protein, 4.5g carbohydrates, 11.5g fat

YOGURT PARFAIT

SERVINGS: 4 **MAKES: ABOUT 2 CUPS** **TIME: 2 HOURS 15 MIN (OVERNIGHT)**

INGREDIENTS:

1/4 cup rolled oats
1/4 cup unsweetened almond or coconut milk
1 scoop chocolate protein powder
5.3 ounce container vanilla or coconut yogurt
1 banana, mashed with a fork

- PUREED DIET
- SOFT FOODS DIET
- GENERAL DIET

DIRECTIONS:

1. Combine oats and almond or coconut milk in a mason jar, stirring until oats are submerged in the liquid. Place in the refrigerator for two hours or overnight.
2. In a small food processor or blender, blend together oat mixture and protein powder until a pureed texture.
3. In four small mason jars layer 1/4 cup yogurt, 1/4 mashed banana, and 1/4 of the oat mixture.
4. You can top with cinnamon, a little drizzle of honey, or eat it just as it is!

Nutrition Facts (1/4 of recipe):
98 calories, 11g protein, 11g carbohydrates, 1g fat

MASHED CAULIFLOWER

SERVINGS: 3   MAKES: 1 1/2 CUPS   TIME: 10 MINUTES

INGREDIENTS:

3 cup cauliflower florets, chopped and steamed
2 TBSP Parmesan cheese
1 TBSP asiago cheese
1 tsp butter
1/2 TBSP sour cream
1/2 TBSP half-and-half milk
1/4 tsp salt
1/4 tsp pepper
1/2 tsp garlic powder

Optional ingredient:
1 scoop unflavored protein powder

DIRECTIONS:

1. Combine cauliflower, Parmesan cheese, asiago cheese, butter, sour cream, half-and-half, salt, pepper, and garlic powder in a blender. Blend on high until a smooth consistency.
2. Carefully remove mashed cauliflower from the blender and transfer into a small bowl. Portion out 1/2 cup and add 1 scoop of protein powder if desired. Do not add protein powder until ready to eat.

- PUREED DIET
- SOFT FOODS DIET
- GENERAL DIET

Nutrition Facts (1/2 cup + 1 scoop protein powder):
160 calories, 25g protein, 5g carbohydrates, 4g fat

APPLE CINNAMON OATMEAL

SERVINGS: 4   MAKES: ABOUT 2 CUPS   TIME: 15 MINUTES

INGREDIENTS:

1/2 cup rolled oats
1/2 cup 1% milk
1 scoop vanilla protein powder
1/2 cup unsweetened applesauce
Cinnamon

- PUREED DIET
- SOFT FOODS DIET
- GENERAL DIET

DIRECTIONS:

1. Combine oats and milk, cook according to package instructions. Alternatively you can combine the oats and milk in a mason jar and leave in the refrigerator for two hours or overnight.
2. Transfer oat and milk mixture to a small food processor or blender and add protein powder; blend together until a smooth consistency.
3. In four small mason jars layer 1/4 cup oat and protein mixture, 2 TBSP applesauce, and sprinkle each with cinnamon to taste.

Nutrition Facts (1/4 of recipe):
88 calories, 7g protein, 11g carbohydrates, 1g fat

Part Three: Pureed Foods

PB & J OVERNIGHT OATS

SERVINGS: 1   **MAKES:** 1/2-3/4 CUP   **TIME:** 2 HOURS 15 MIN (OVERNIGHT)

INGREDIENTS:

2 TBSP rolled oats
1/4 unsweetened almond milk
1 TBSP powdered peanut butter
1/2 scoop vanilla protein powder
1/4 cup frozen raspberries
1 tsp pure maple syrup
1 tsp half-and-half milk

Optional topping:
1 tsp creamy peanut butter

DIRECTIONS:

1. In a small mason jar combine the rolled oats and almond milk. Refrigerate and let the oats soak for at least two hours or overnight.
2. Empty the oats and almond milk mixture into a small blender or food processor; add powdered peanut butter and protein powder. Blend until a pureed texture.
3. Transfer the pureed oat mixture back into the mason jar and set aside. Rinse out the blender/food processor.
4. Add the frozen raspberries, maple syrup and half-and-half to the food processor. Blend until a pureed texture; the raspberry mixture should resemble the texture and appearance of a fruit sorbet.
5. Top the oat mixture with the raspberry sorbet and you have the option of drizzling with a small amount of creamy peanut butter.

- PUREED DIET
- SOFT FOODS DIET
- GENERAL DIET

Nutrition Facts (without peanut butter drizzle):
156 calories, 14.5g protein, 17g carbohydrates, 2.5g fat

TIPS/SUGGESTIONS:
- Make multiple servings and portion into small mason jars for an easy breakfast or snack during the day.
- If preparing ahead of time, separate the oat mixture and raspberries in separate containers until ready to eat.

SPRING THYME VEGETABLE SOUP

SERVINGS: 5 **MAKES: 2 1/2 CUPS** **TIME: 35 MINUTES**

INGREDIENTS:

1 tsp olive oil
1/2 cup yellow onion, chopped
4 cloves garlic, minced
1/2 small summer squash, chopped
1/2 large zucchini, chopped
1/2 cup celery, chopped
1 1/2 cup vegetable broth
1/2 15 ounce can cannellini beans, drained and rinsed
1/2 tsp salt
1/2 tsp pepper
1 tsp fresh thyme leaves, stems removed and packed

Optional ingredient:
1 scoop unflavored protein powder (per serving)

DIRECTIONS:

1. In a medium-sized pot, preheat olive oil over medium heat on the stove top.
2. Add onion and garlic to the pot, stirring and cooking until fragrant, about 2 minutes.
3. Add summer squash, zucchini and celery to the pot. Cook until vegetables begin to soften, about 3-4 minutes.
4. Add the vegetable broth to the pot and bring to a boil. Add the cannellini beans, salt, pepper, and thyme. Return the pot to a boil, cover and reduce heat. Simmer on low for 20 minutes.
5. Remove pot from the heat and uncover; allow the soup to cool for 5 minutes.
6. Transfer soup to a blender or food processor and pulse 3-4 times to create a pureed texture.
7. Portion out soup and allow to cool down to 140 degrees F, mix in 1 scoop protein powder if desired but don't include protein powder until you are ready to eat the soup.

- PUREED DIET
- SOFT FOODS DIET
- GENERAL DIET

Nutrition Facts (1/2 cup soup + 1 scoop protein powder): 155 calories, 24g protein, 11g carbohydrates, 1g fat

TIPS/SUGGESTIONS:
- To make this soup ahead of time, portion into small containers and refrigerate for up to two to three days.
- Not on a pureed diet? Skip the blender step and enjoy this soup on a soft foods diet or general diet and add canned chicken for more protein.

Part Three: Pureed Foods

VEGETABLE CHILI

SERVINGS: 4-5   **MAKES:** 2-2 1/2 CUPS   **TIME:** 40 MINUTES

INGREDIENTS:

1 tsp olive oil
3 cloves garlic
1/2 cup yellow onion, chopped
1/2 cup shredded carrots
1/2 cup bell pepper, chopped
1 cup cauliflower, chopped
1/4 cup corn
1/4 cup canned green chiles
1/2 14.5 ounce can diced tomatoes (with their juice)
2 cups broth
1/2 tsp salt
1 TBSP chili powder
1 tsp cumin
1/4 tsp paprika
1/2 15 ounce can pinto beans, drained and rinsed

Optional ingredients:
1/2-1 scoop unflavored protein powder
1/2 TBSP sour cream or plain Greek yogurt

- PUREED DIET
- SOFT FOODS DIET
- GENERAL DIET

DIRECTIONS:

1. Preheat olive oil in a medium-sized pot over medium heat on the stove top.
2. Add the garlic and stir for about 1 minute. Add the onion, carrots, bell pepper, cauliflower, and corn to the pot. Stir and let the vegetables cook for 2-3 minutes while stirring occasionally.
3. Add the green chiles and diced tomatoes; stir until well combined.
4. Add the broth, salt, chili powder, cumin, paprika, and pinto beans to the pot. Bring to a boil then reduce heat to low and simmer for 20 minutes.
5. Remove from heat and let it cool for about 5 minutes.
6. Transfer soup to a blender and pulse 3-4 times to create a pureed texture.
7. Portion out 1/2 cup, let it cool to 140 degrees F and stir in protein powder if desired. Don't include protein powder until ready to eat. Top with a dollop of sour cream or plain Greek yogurt for a creamy topping if you would like (not included in calories below).

Nutrition Facts (1/2 cup + 1 scoop protein powder):
180 calories, 24g protein, 17g carbohydrates, 1g fat

TIPS/SUGGESTIONS:
- To make this soup ahead of time, portion into small containers and refrigerate for up to two to three days.
- Not on a pureed diet? Skip the blender step and enjoy this soup on a soft foods diet or general diet.

WHITE BEAN CHILI VERDE

SERVINGS: 5　　**MAKES:** 2 1/2 CUPS　　**TIME:** 25 MINUTES

INGREDIENTS:

1 tsp olive oil
1/3 cup white onion, diced
1/2 4 ounce can green chiles
1/4 cup salsa verde (green salsa)
5 ounce can of chicken breast
1/4 tsp salt
3 cloves garlic, minced
1/4 tsp cumin
1/2 14 ounce can cannellini beans
1 cup chicken broth

Optional ingredients:
Red pepper flakes
Dollop of sour cream

DIRECTIONS:

1. Preheat olive oil in a medium-sized pot over medium heat on the stove top.
2. Add onion and green chiles, while stirring occasionally. Cook until the onions begin to soften, about 3-4 minutes.
3. Add salsa verde, canned chicken, salt, garlic, cumin and beans to the pot. Stir well and continue to stir until mixture comes to a boil.
4. Add chicken broth and bring soup to a boil. Reduce heat to low, cover and let the soup simmer for 10 minutes.
5. Remove pot from the heat and let it cool for 5 minutes. Transfer soup to a blender or food processor, pulse 4-5 times to create a pureed texture.
6. Top with a dollop of sour cream if you would like, or if you want additional spice include some red pepper flakes.

- PUREED DIET
- SOFT FOODS DIET
- GENERAL DIET

Nutrition Facts (1/2 cup):
87 calories, 9g protein, 11g carbohydrates, 1.5g fat

TIPS/SUGGESTIONS:
- To make this soup ahead of time, portion into small containers and refrigerate for up to two to three days.
- Not on a pureed diet? Skip the blender step and enjoy this soup on a soft foods diet or general diet.

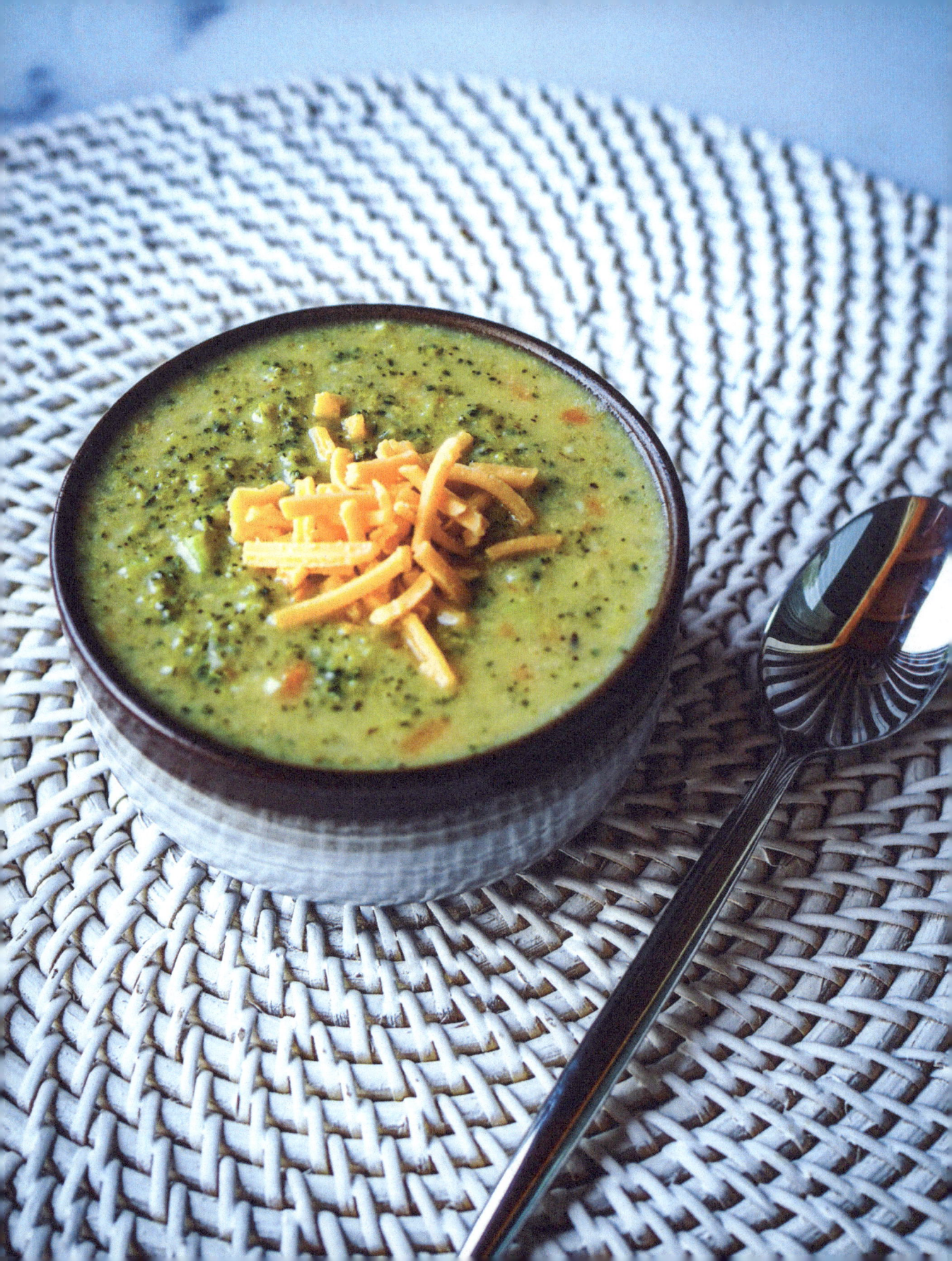

BROCCOLI CHEDDAR SOUP

SERVINGS: 4   **MAKES: 2 CUPS**   **TIME: 45 MINUTES**

INGREDIENTS:

1 tsp olive oil
1/4 cup onion, diced
1/4 cup shredded carrots
2 cups broccoli florets, chopped
2 cloves garlic, minced
1 cup chicken broth
1/4 tsp salt
1/4 tsp pepper
1/4 tsp oregano
1 pinch cayenne pepper
1/4 cup 1% milk
1/2 cup shredded cheddar cheese
1 TBSP nutritional yeast
2 tsp corn starch

Optional ingredient:
1/2-1 scoop unflavored protein powder

DIRECTIONS:

1. Preheat olive oil over medium heat in a medium pot on the stove top.
2. Add onion, carrots, broccoli and garlic to the pot, stir well. Cook until the vegetables begin to soften, about 6 minutes while stirring occasionally.
3. Add chicken broth, salt, pepper, oregano, and cayenne pepper to the pot and bring to a boil. Reduce the heat to low, cover, and let it simmer for about 10 minutes or until the broccoli becomes very soft.
4. Remove soup from the heat and let it cool for 5 minutes.
5. Transfer soup to a blender or food processor and pulse 4-5 times to create a pureed texture.
6. Return the soup to the pot and put it back over low heat on the stove top.
7. Slowly stir in milk, cheddar cheese, and nutritional yeast. Continuing to stir frequently, bring to a low boil, and then remove from the heat. It's important not to use a higher heat during this phase so you don't burn the milk.
8. After removing pot from the heat, stir in corn starch and make sure it is well combined and free of lumps. Let it cool for about 6 minutes to let it thicken. Yum!
9. If including protein powder portion out 1/2 cup and allow to cool to 140 degrees F before mixing in this optional ingredient.

- PUREED DIET
- SOFT FOODS DIET
- GENERAL DIET

Nutrition Facts (1/2 cup):
105 calories, 7g protein, 9g carbohydrates, 6g fat

TIPS/SUGGESTIONS:
- To make this soup ahead of time, portion into small containers and refrigerate for up to two to three days.
- Not on a pureed diet? Skip the blender step and enjoy this soup on a soft foods diet or general diet.

Part Four: Fruit Smoothies

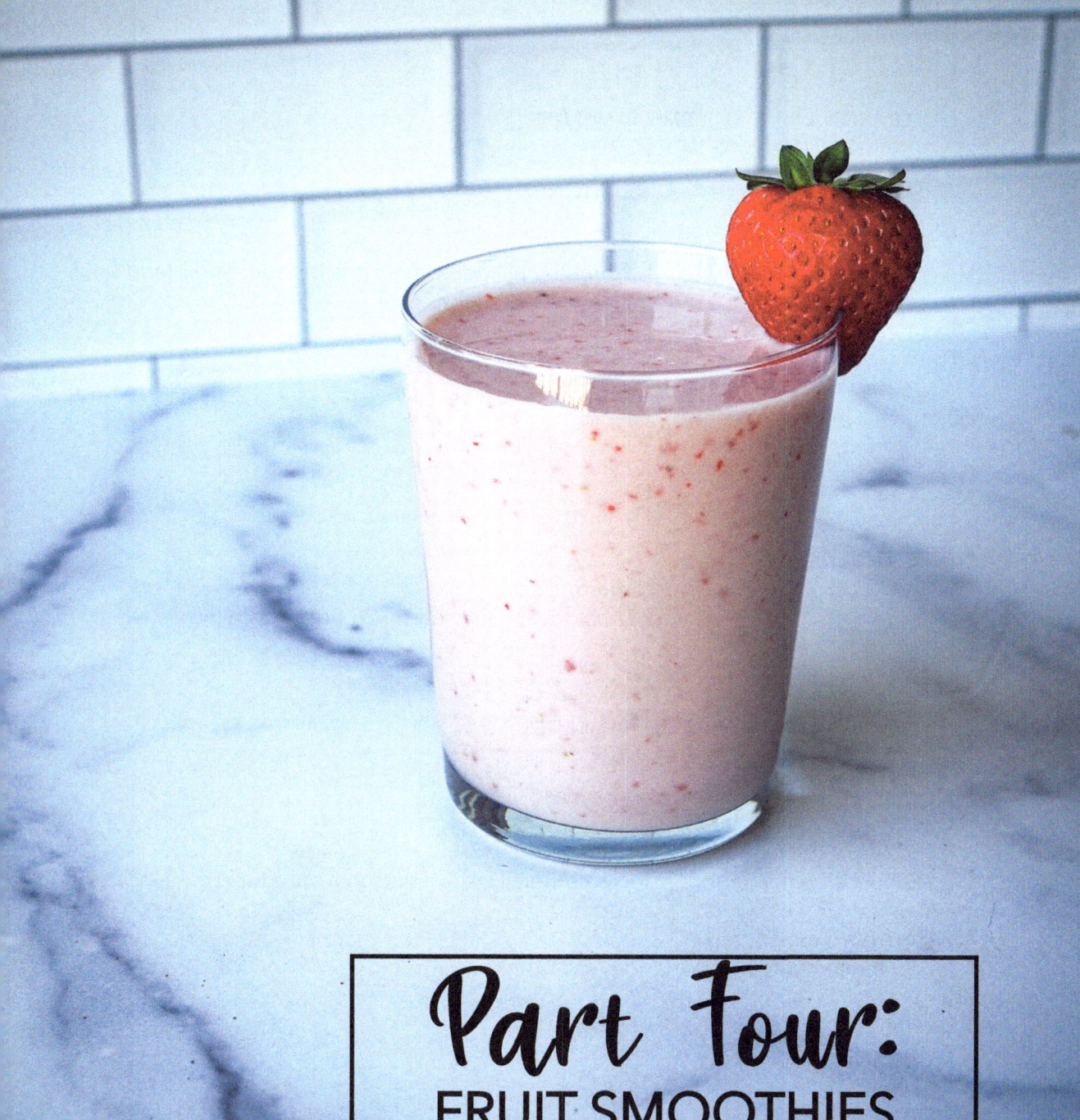

Part Four:
FRUIT SMOOTHIES

Part Four: Fruit Smoothies

GREEN SMOOTHIE

SERVINGS: 1 **TIME:** 10 MINUTES

INGREDIENTS:

1/4 cup spinach, packed
1/4 banana
1/4 cup frozen pineapple
2 TBSP avocado
1/4 cup pear, diced
5.3 ounce container low fat Greek yogurt, plain or vanilla
1 cup cold water

- PUREED DIET
- SOFT FOODS DIET
- GENERAL DIET

DIRECTIONS:

1. Combine all ingredients in a blender and blend until smooth.

Nutrition Facts:
207 calories, 13g protein, 28.5g carbohydrates, 6g fat

WILD BERRY SMOOTHIE

SERVINGS: 1 **TIME:** 10 MINUTES

INGREDIENTS:

1/2 5.3 ounce container plain low fat Greek yogurt
1/2 cup frozen mixed berries
1 scoop vanilla protein powder
1 tsp honey
1/2 cup unsweetened almond milk
1/2 cup cold water

- PUREED DIET
- SOFT FOODS DIET
- GENERAL DIET

DIRECTIONS:

1. Combine all ingredients in a blender and blend until smooth.

Nutrition Facts:
208 calories, 25.5g protein, 18g carbohydrates, 3.5g fat

PEANUT BUTTER BANANA SMOOTHIE

SERVINGS: 1   **TIME: 10 MINUTES**

INGREDIENTS:

5.3 ounce container vanilla low fat Greek yogurt
1 TBSP peanut butter
1 TBSP powdered peanut butter
1/2 banana
1/2 cup unsweetened almond milk
1/2 cup cold water

- PUREED DIET
- SOFT FOODS DIET
- GENERAL DIET

DIRECTIONS:

1. Combine all ingredients in a blender and blend until smooth.

Nutrition Facts:
266 calories, 20.5g protein, 21.5g carbohydrates, 12g fat

PINEAPPLE MANGO SMOOTHIE

SERVINGS: 1   **TIME: 10 MINUTES**

INGREDIENTS:

5.3 ounce container coconut low fat Greek yogurt
1/4 cup frozen pineapple
1/4 cup frozen mango
1 cup cold water
1/4 banana

- PUREED DIET
- SOFT FOODS DIET
- GENERAL DIET

DIRECTIONS:

1. Combine all ingredients in a blender and blend until smooth.

Nutrition Facts:
179 calories, 13.5 protein, 27g carbohydrates, 2g fat

Part Four: Fruit Smoothies

STRAWBERRY BANANA SMOOTHIE

SERVINGS: 1   **TIME:** 10 MINUTES

INGREDIENTS:

2-4 ice cubes
4 strawberries, stems removed
5.3 ounce container strawberry low fat Greek yogurt
1/2 banana
1 cup unsweetened vanilla almond milk

- PUREED DIET
- SOFT FOODS DIET
- GENERAL DIET

DIRECTIONS:

1. Combine all ingredients in a blender and blend until smooth.

Nutrition Facts:
198 calories, 15g protein, 26g carbohydrates, 4g fat

BLUEBERRY PIE SMOOTHIE

SERVINGS: 1   **TIME:** 10 MINUTES

INGREDIENTS:

5.3 ounce container vanilla low fat Greek yogurt
1/3 cup fresh blueberries
1/4 tsp cinnamon
1 tsp pure maple syrup
2 TBSP rolled oats
1 cup unsweetened oat milk

- PUREED DIET
- SOFT FOODS DIET
- GENERAL DIET

DIRECTIONS:

1. Combine all ingredients in a blender and blend until smooth.

Nutrition Facts:
235 calories, 15g protein, 30g carbohydrates, 6g fat

Part Five:
BREAKFAST

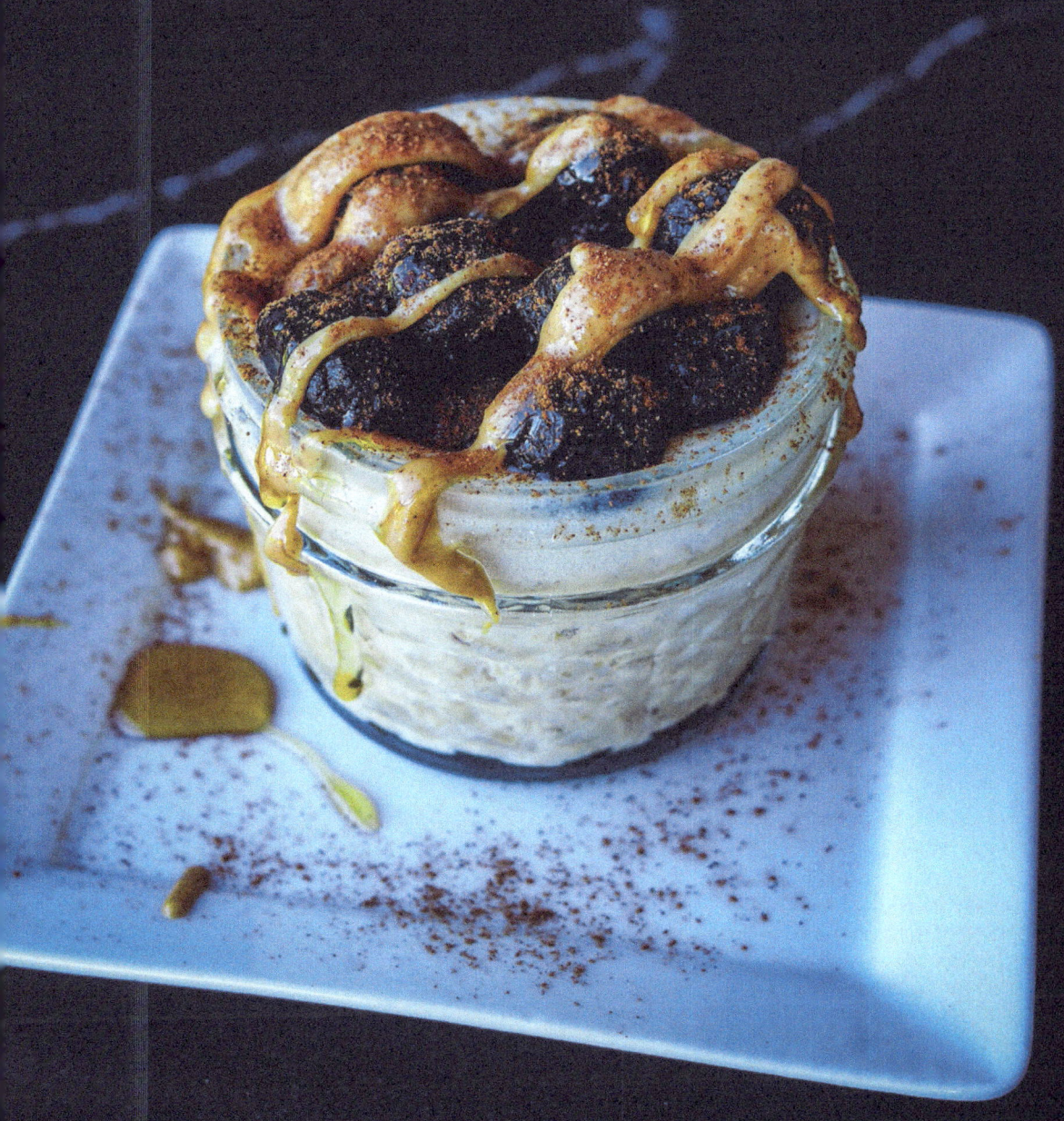

Part Five: Breakfast

SWEET POTATO VEGETABLE HASH

SERVINGS: 3   **MAKES: 1 1/2 CUPS**   **TIME: 30 MINUTES**

INGREDIENTS:

1 tsp olive oil
1/2 cup sweet potato, peeled and diced
1/4 cup celery, diced
2 TBSP onion, peeled and diced
1/4 cup asparagus, diced
1 chicken sausage link, diced
1/8 tsp salt
1/8 tsp pepper
1/8 tsp sage
1/8 tsp thyme

Optional topping:
1 egg
1 TBSP green onion, diced

DIRECTIONS:

1. Preheat oil in a large pan over medium-high heat on stove top.
2. Once heated, add the sweet potatoes and stir until well coated with oil. Cover the pan and let it cook for 8-10 minutes, stirring occasionally to prevent potatoes from sticking to the pan.
3. Uncover the pan and add celery, onion, and asparagus. Cover the pan and let it continue cooking for 6 minutes, stirring occasionally.
4. Add chicken sausage, salt, pepper, sage, and thyme. Stir until well combined and cover. Cook for another 5-7 minutes.
5. Uncover, remove from heat, and top with an egg and green onion.

● **GENERAL DIET**

Nutrition Facts (1/2 cup hash + 1 egg):
219 calories, 13g protein, 13g carbohydrates, 13g fat

TIPS/SUGGESTIONS:
1. Additional optional toppings include hot sauce, avocado, and Parmesan cheese.
2. Double this recipe, portion into plastic containers; include 1 hard-boiled egg in each container and have breakfast for the week.

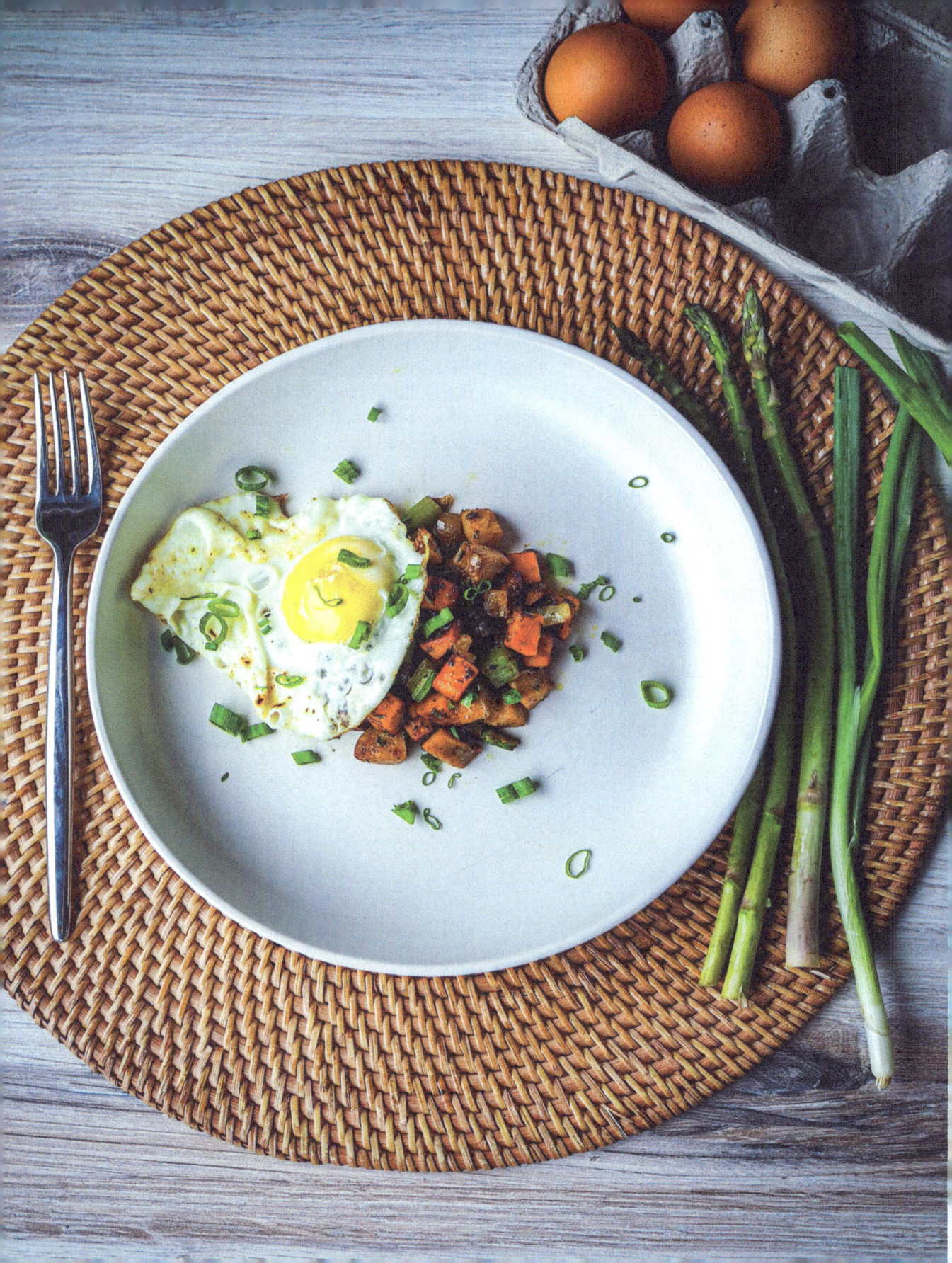

Part Five: Breakfast

MEDITERRANEAN FRITTATA

SERVINGS: 2　　**MAKES: 2 FRITTATAS**　　**TIME: 30 MINUTES**

INGREDIENTS:

1 tsp olive oil
1 handful spinach
2 cloves garlic, minced
1 egg
2 egg whites
1 TBSP half-and-half milk
1/8 tsp salt
1/8 tsp pepper
1 TBSP feta cheese, crumbled
1/8 tsp dried thyme
1/8 tsp dried sage
4 cherry tomatoes, sliced in half
1 TBSP green onion, diced
2 tsp balsamic glaze

DIRECTIONS:

1. Preheat oven to 400 degrees F.
2. Heat a small cast iron skillet over medium heat on stove top, add garlic and spinach, saute until spinach is wilted, then take the skillet off the heat and set aside.
3. While the skillet is cooling down add the egg, egg whites, half-and-half, salt, pepper, feta cheese, thyme, and sage to a small bowl. Whisk with a fork until well combined.
4. Add egg mixture to the cast iron skillet and bake in the oven for 14 minutes, or until cooked through.
5. Take the skillet out of the oven and turn up the oven to high broil.
6. Top the frittata with cherry tomatoes and place the skillet back into the oven. Broil on high for 2 minutes.
7. Take the skillet out of the oven, drizzle with balsamic glaze, and sprinkle with green onion.

● **GENERAL DIET**

Nutrition Facts (1/2 recipe):
115 calories, 8g protein, 5g carbohydrates, 6.5g fat

TIPS/SUGGESTIONS:
- Add additional vegetable toppings to increase your dietary fiber and increase feelings of fullness if needed.
- Instead of balsamic glaze, you can top with a small amount of basil pesto to add great flavor.

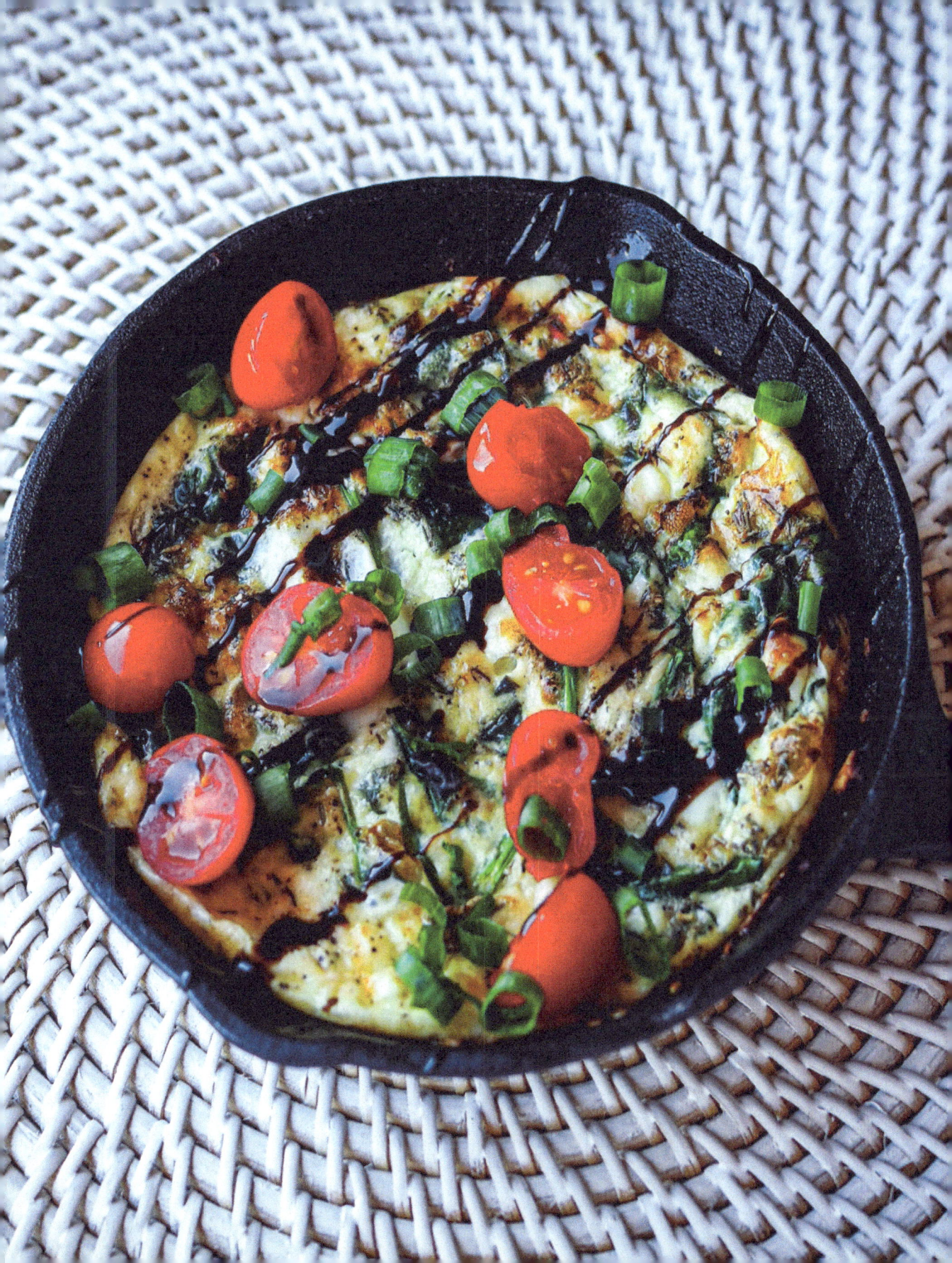

Part Five: Breakfast

PEANUT BUTTER PROTEIN BOMBS

SERVINGS: 3 **MAKES: 6 BOMBS** **TIME: 10 MINUTES**

INGREDIENTS:

1 scoop chocolate protein powder
1/4 cup almond flour
2 TBSP creamy peanut butter
2 TBSP dark chocolate chips
2 tsp honey
1 TBSP hemp hearts
2 TBSP powdered peanut butter
1-2 TBSP unsweetened vanilla almond milk

● GENERAL DIET

DIRECTIONS:

1. In a medium-sized mixing bowl combine the protein powder, almond flour, peanut butter, chocolate chips, honey, hemp hearts, and powdered peanut butter.
2. The mixture should be pretty dry. Slowly start to add in almond milk, 1 TBSP at a time until the mixture begins to clump and it sticks together easily. Be careful not to add too much almond milk to prevent from mixture getting too wet.
3. Divide the mixture into 6 portions and form into small balls. Store in an airtight container in the refrigerator until you are ready to eat.

Nutrition Facts (for 2 bombs):
244 calories, 13g protein, 16g carbohydrates, 15g fat

CHIA SEED PUDDING

SERVINGS: 2-3 **MAKES: 1 1/2 CUPS** **TIME: 7-8 HOURS (OVERNIGHT)**

INGREDIENTS:

1 scoop vanilla protein powder
1 cup 1% milk
2 TBSP chia seeds
1 banana, sliced
2 TBSP creamy peanut butter

● SOFT FOODS DIET
● GENERAL DIET

DIRECTIONS:

1. Using a milk frother or shaker bottle, mix together the milk and protein powder until a smooth texture.
2. Using 2 small mason jars (or other container), mix together 1 TBSP chia seeds and half of the milk mixture in each jar. Cover with a lid and place in the refrigerator overnight.
3. In the morning when you are ready to eat, top with 1/2 sliced banana and 1 TBSP peanut butter. It's normal for the mixture to separate overnight while soaking, just give it a good stir before adding the toppings.
4. This is a great recipe to prep on the weekends to have breakfast ready for the week!

Nutrition Facts (1/2 of recipe):
276 calories, 20g protein, 28g carbohydrates, 11g fat

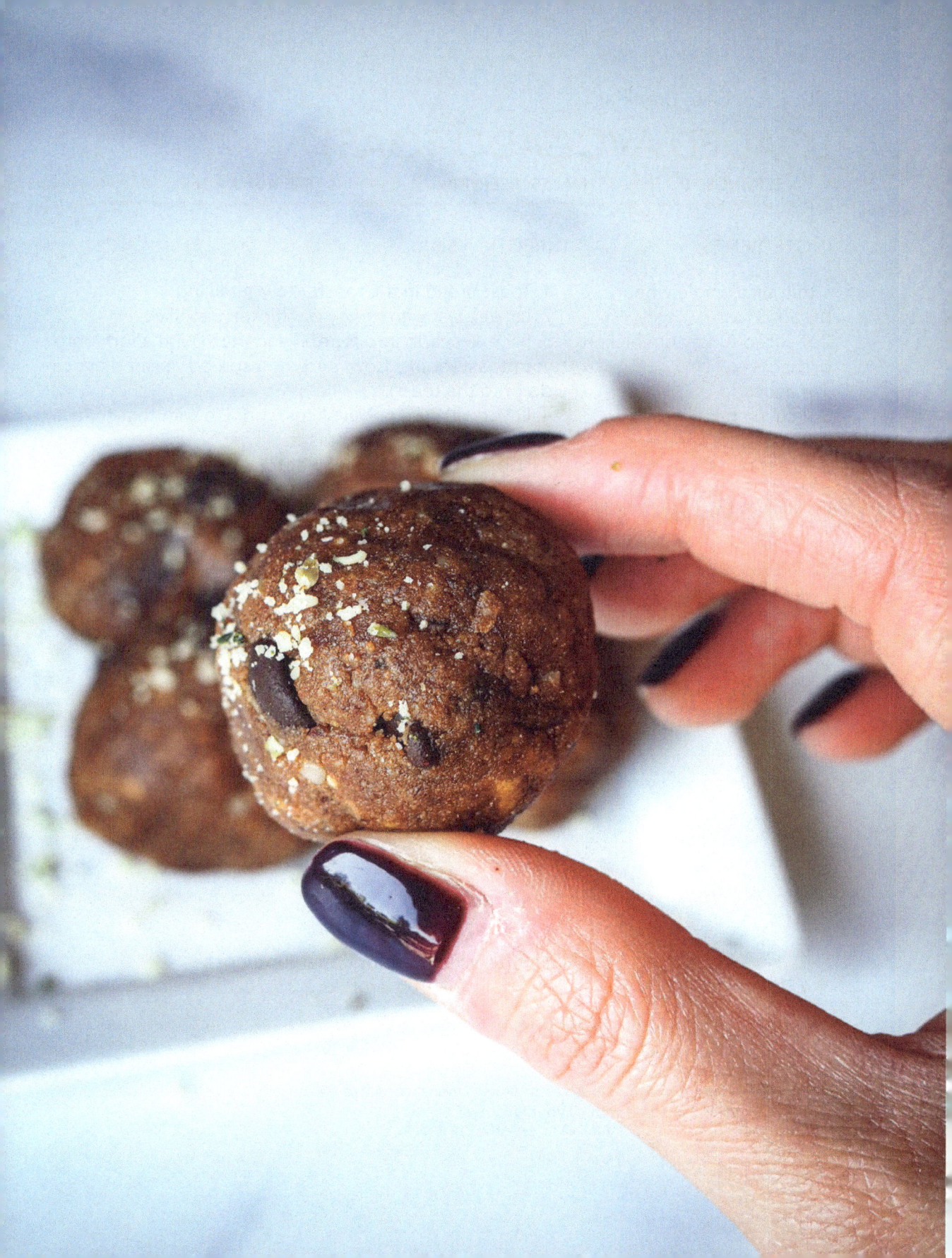

Part Five: Breakfast
LOADED AVOCADO TOAST

SERVINGS: 1 **MAKES: 1 SERVING** **TIME: 10 MINUTES**

INGREDIENTS:

1 thin slice whole wheat bread
2oz sliced turkey or chicken breast
1/4 avocado
3-4 cucumber slices
1-2 TBSP feta cheese
Salt/pepper, to taste

Optional toppings:
Chia Seeds
Sprouts
Hot sauce
Hemp hearts
Lemon Juice
Fresh herbs
Shredded carrots
Spinach

DIRECTIONS:

1. Toast bread in the toaster to your liking.
2. Layer toast with turkey or chicken deli slices.
3. Slice avocado into fourths and mash with a fork onto your toast (or in a bowl and then spread mashed avocado onto the toast).
4. Layer with cucumber slices, sprinkle with feta cheese, and add salt/pepper to taste.
6. Top with tomato and other toppings as desired.

This recipes makes a great breakfast or snack. It is quick and easy to throw together in a hurry and very nutrient dense!

● **GENERAL DIET**

Nutrition Facts (no optional toppings):
241 calories, 18g protein, 21.5g carbohydrates, 11g fat

TIPS/SUGGESTIONS:
- If you are needing a higher protein content, mix unflavored protein powder with mashed avocado
- Get creative with this recipe; there are no rules when it comes to avocado toast, so load it up with all your favorites!

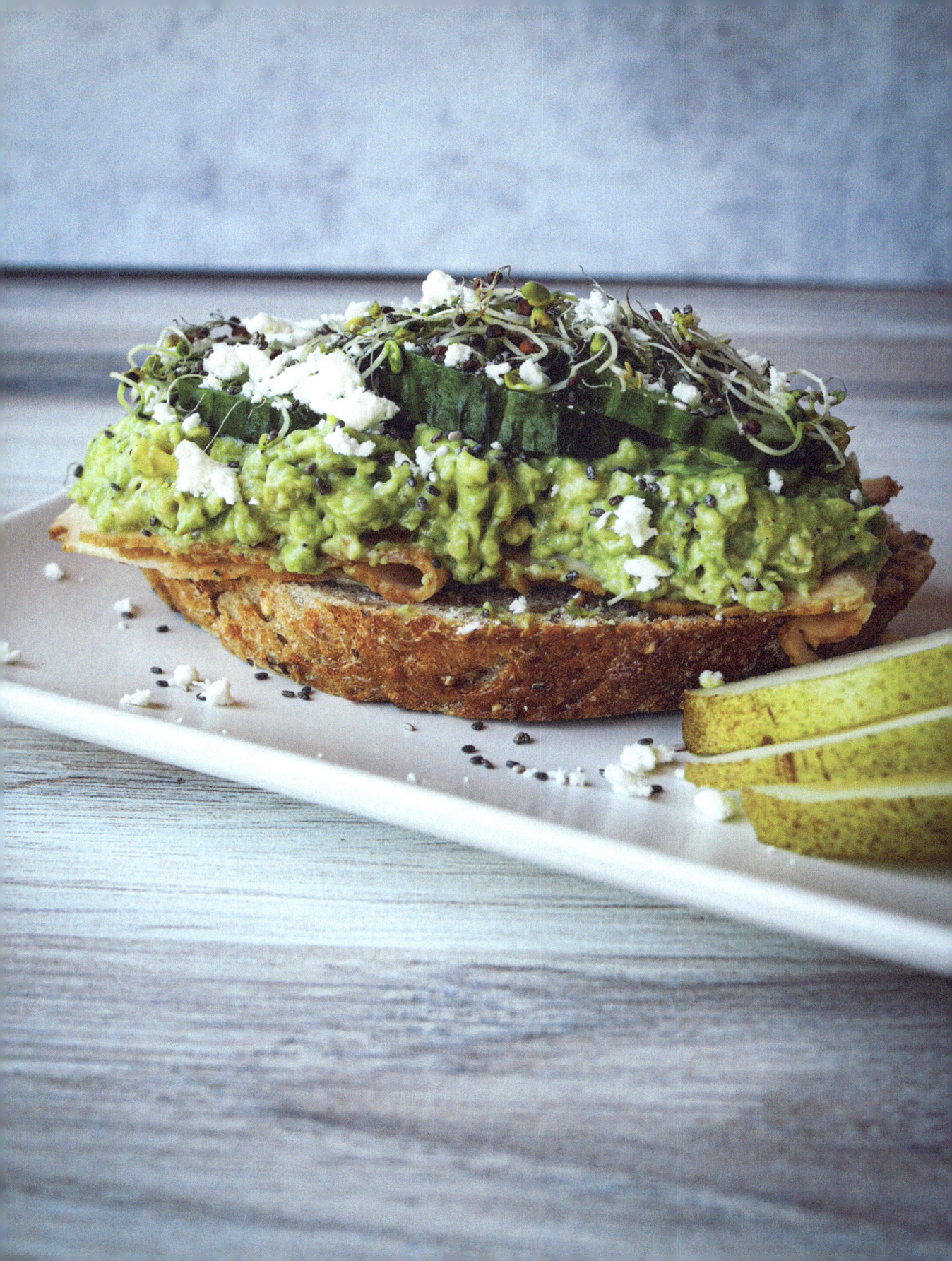

Part Five: Breakfast

OVERNIGHT OATS

SERVINGS: 1   **MAKES: 1 SERVING**   **TIME: 2 HOURS 25 MIN (OVERNIGHT)**

INGREDIENTS:

1/2 cup unsweetened vanilla almond milk
1 scoop vanilla protein powder
1/4 cup oats
1/4 cup blueberries, fresh or frozen
1 TBSP peanut butter
Pinch of cinnamon

DIRECTIONS:

1. Add almond milk and protein powder to a large cup and use a milk frother or shaker bottle to blend the ingredients until smooth.
2. Add oats and almond milk mixture to a small mason jar (or other container), stir well, and cover tightly with a lid. Place in the refrigerator for two hours or up to two days.
3. Remove from the refrigerator, top with blueberries, peanut butter and cinnamon. Enjoy!

- SOFT FOODS DIET
- GENERAL DIET

Nutrition Facts:
306 calories, 26g protein, 26g carbohydrates, 12g fat

TIPS/SUGGESTIONS:
1. If you are trying to decrease calories you can use powdered peanut butter instead of creamy peanut butter.

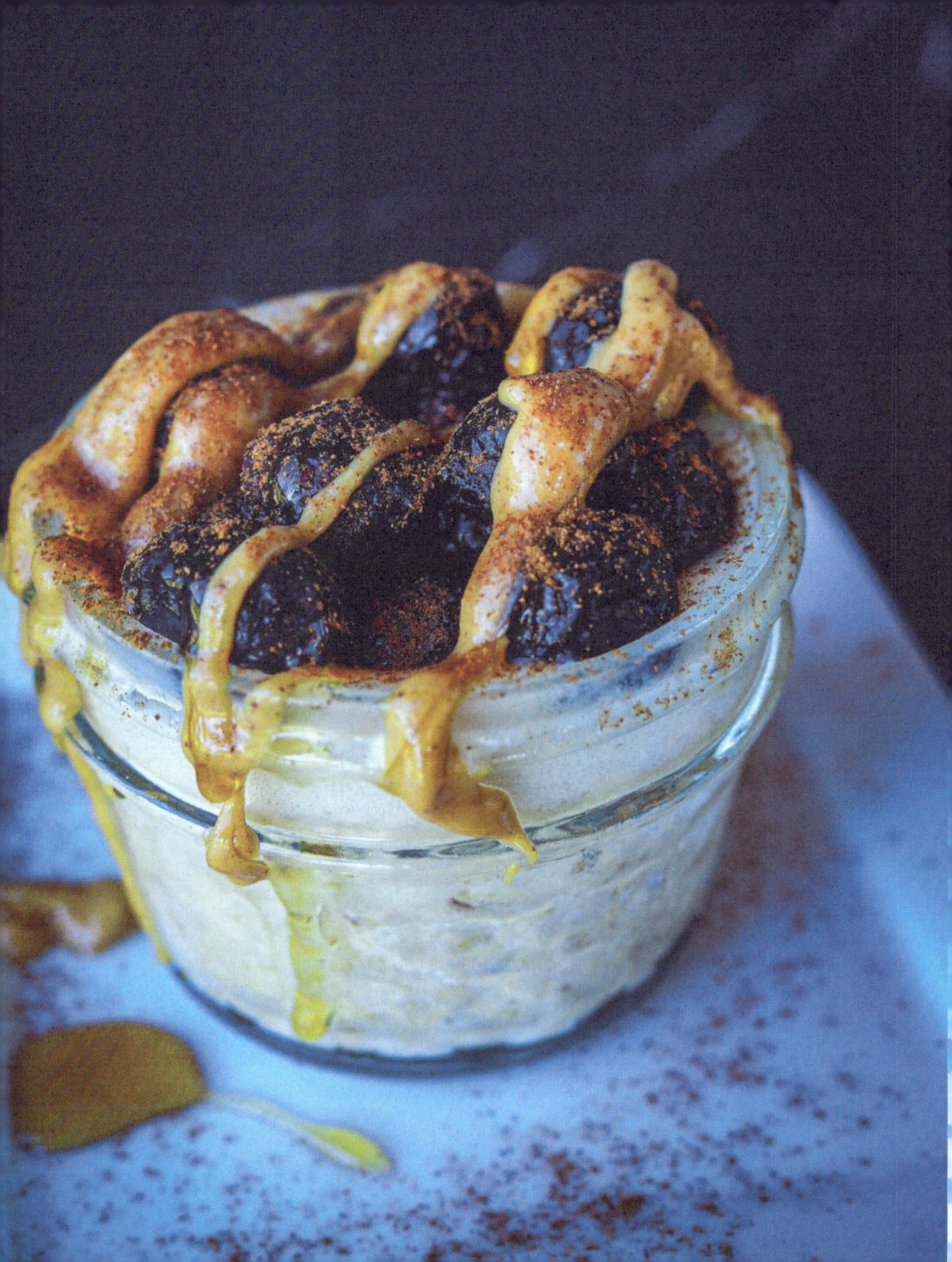

Part Five: Breakfast

BACON CHEDDAR CHAFFLE

SERVINGS: 2 **MAKES: 1 LARGE CHAFFLE** **TIME: 20 MINUTES**

INGREDIENTS:

2 slices bacon, diced
1 egg
1/4 cup shredded cheddar cheese
1 TBSP almond flour
1/4 tsp baking powder
1/4 tsp garlic powder
Salt/pepper to taste

DIRECTIONS:

1. Preheat a small pan over medium heat on the stove top. Also preheat a small waffle iron.
2. Add bacon to the pan and cook until brown and cooked through, about 5-minutes per side.
3. Remove pan from the heat, drain excess fat from the pan, and discard. Allow the bacon to cool for about 5 minutes.
4. In a small bowl combine egg, cheddar cheese, almond flour, baking powder, and garlic powder. Whisk with a fork until well combined and stir in cooked bacon. Salt and pepper to taste.
5. Pour mixture into the waffle iron and cook until lightly browned, about 2-3 minutes. Remove from the waffle iron and enjoy!

● **GENERAL DIET**

Nutrition Facts (1/2 recipe):
159 calories, 10.5g protein, 1g carbohydrates, 11.5g fat

TIPS/SUGGESTIONS:
- Pair half of this recipe with a serving of fruit for a healthy dose of fiber and carbohydrates.

SAUSAGE CHAFFLE

SERVINGS: 2   **MAKES: 1 LARGE CHAFFLE**   **TIME: 20 MINUTES**

INGREDIENTS:

4 ounces ground turkey sausage
2 TBSP salsa verde
1 egg
1/4 cup shredded mozzarella cheese
1 TBSP almond flour
1/4 tsp baking powder
1/4 tsp garlic powder
Pinch of salt

Optional topping:
1 TBSP sour cream
1 TBSP mashed avocado

DIRECTIONS:

1. Preheat a small pan over medium heat on the stove top. Also preheat a small waffle iron.
2. Add turkey sausage to the pan and cook until browned and cooked through, about 6 minutes. Add salsa verde to the pan and cook until most of the liquid is evaporated, another 3-4 minutes.
3. Remove the pan from the heat and let the mixture cool while you prepare the chaffle base.
4. Combine egg, mozzarella cheese, almond flour, baking powder, garlic powder, and salt in a small bowl; whisk with a fork until well combined. Add the turkey sausage mixture to the bowl and stir well.
5. Pour mixture into the waffle iron and cook until lightly browned, about 2-3 minutes. Remove from the waffle iron and enjoy!
6. If you want to include the topping, mix together sour cream and avocado in a separate small bowl and spread over top of the chaffle.

● GENERAL DIET

Nutrition Facts (1/2 recipe + 1/2 topping):
221 calories, 19g protein, 2g carbohydrates, 14.5g fat

TIPS/SUGGESTIONS:
- Pair half of this recipe with a serving of fruit for a healthy dose of fiber and carbohydrates.

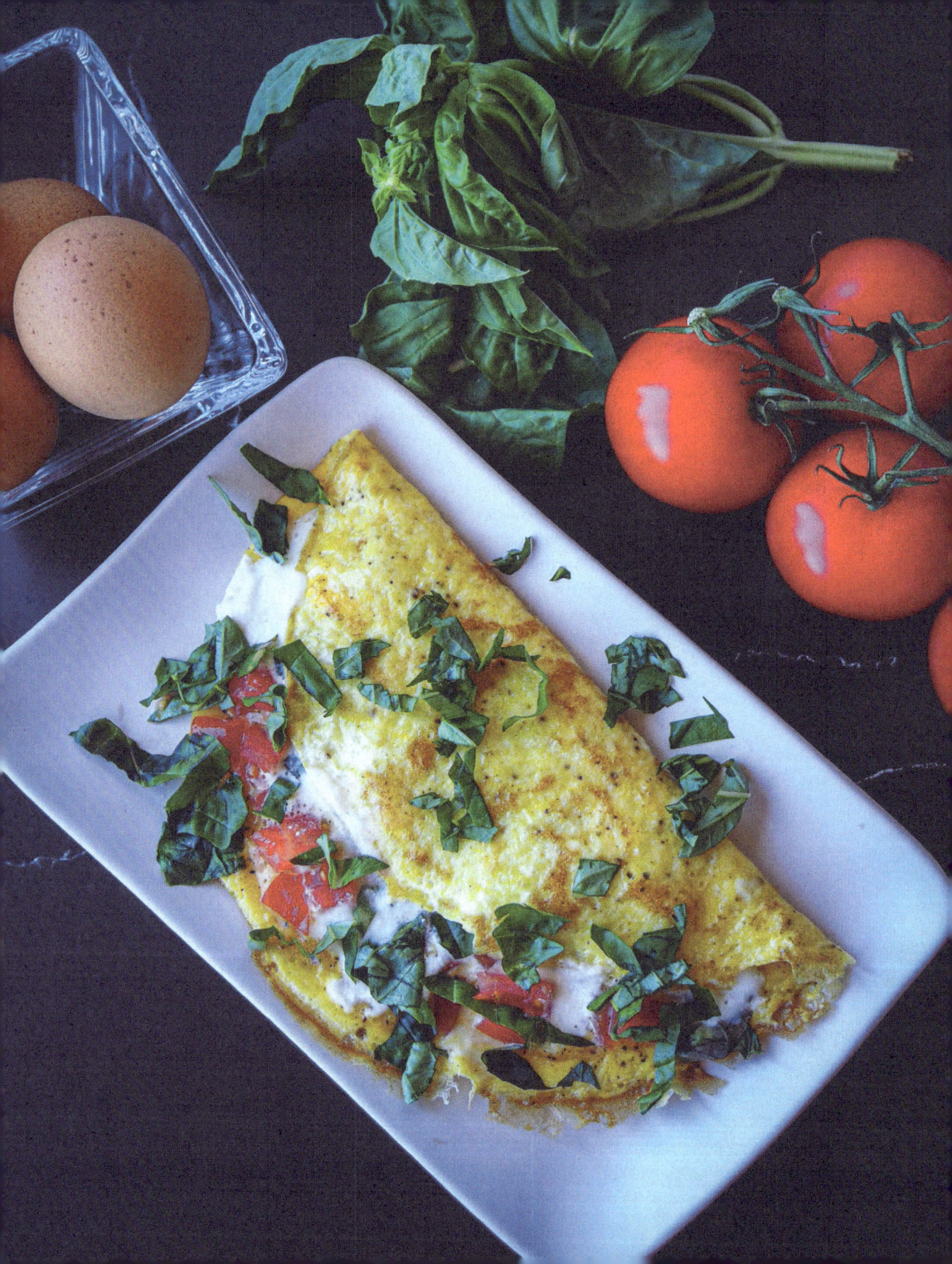

TOMATO BASIL OMELETTE

SERVINGS: 2　　　**MAKES: 2 OMELETTES**　　　**TIME: 15 MINUTES**

INGREDIENTS:

2 eggs
1/8 tsp salt
1/8 tsp pepper
1 TBSP 2% milk
2 TBSP ricotta cheese
1/4 cup tomatoes, diced
1 TBSP fresh basil, sliced thin

DIRECTIONS:

1. Preheat a small nonstick pan over medium-low heat on the stove top and spray with oil.
2. While the pan is preheating, crack 2 eggs into a small bowl. Add salt, pepper and milk, whisk together until well combined.
3. Pour egg mixture into pan and cook for 3-4 minutes. Do not move or disrupt the eggs while they are cooking.
5. Place small dollops of ricotta cheese, diced tomatoes, and 1 TBSP of fresh basil on half the omelette.
4. Carefully take a rubber spatula and run around the edges of the omelette to loosen the omelette from the pan. Flip half the omelette over, remove from heat and cover. Let it sit for 2-4 minutes to finish cooking.
5. Top with additional basil and tomatoes if you would like.

● GENERAL DIET

Nutrition Facts (per 1 omelette):
138 calories, 10g protein, 7g carbohydrates, 9g fat

TIPS/SUGGESTIONS:
- Cook the tomatoes and basil until very soft before adding these ingredients to the omelette and enjoy on a soft foods diet.

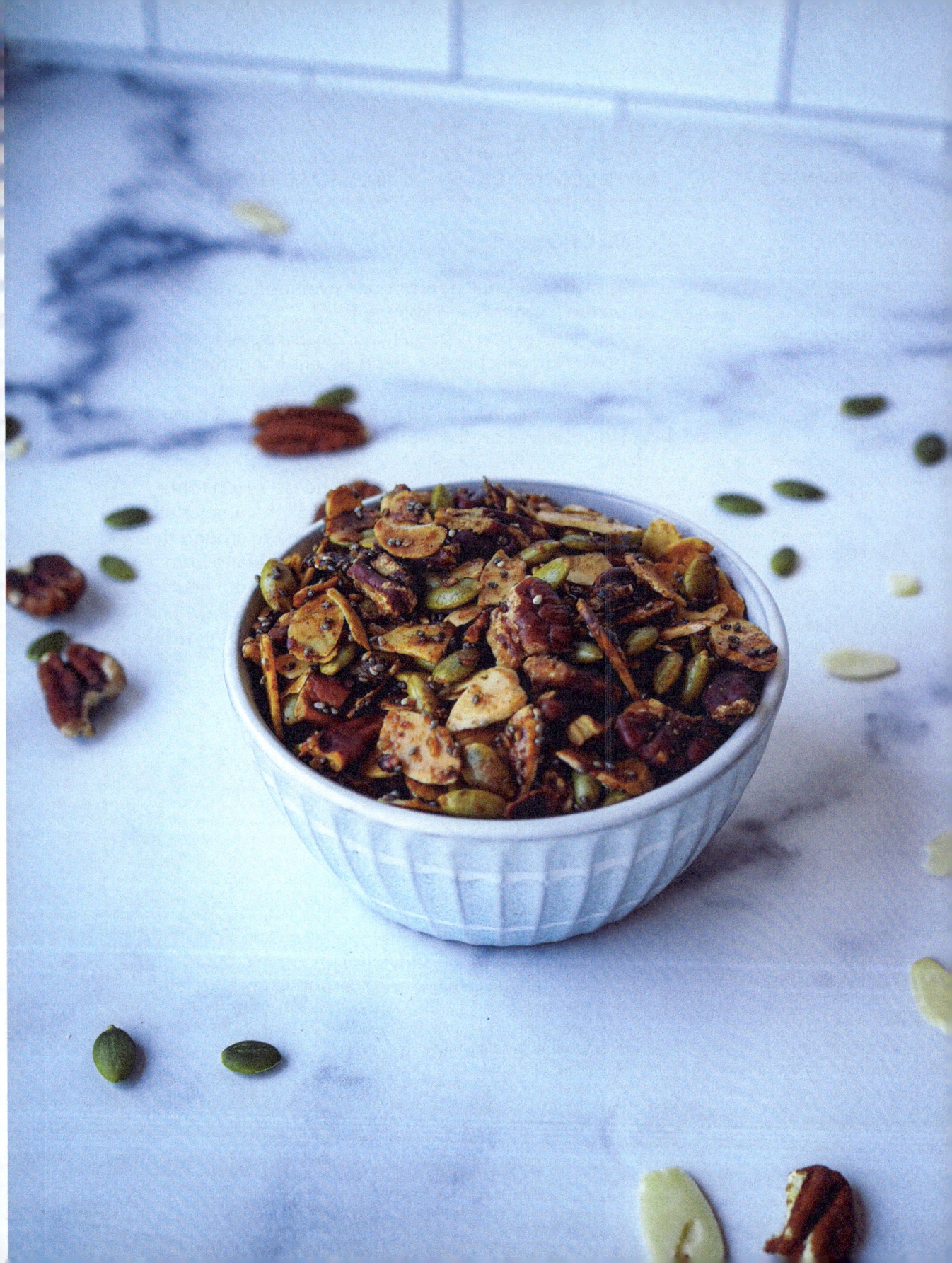

GRAIN-FREE GRANOLA

SERVINGS: 6 **MAKES: 1 1/2 CUPS** **TIME: 22 MINUTES**

INGREDIENTS:

1/2 cup pecans, crushed
1/2 cup sliced almonds
1/4 cup pepitas
1 TBSP chia seeds
1 TBSP pure maple syrup
1 TBSP coconut oil, melted
1/2 tsp ground cinnamon
2 pinches salt

DIRECTIONS:

1. Preheat oven to 400 degrees and line a small baking sheet with tin foil.
2. Combine all ingredients in a medium bowl and stir until well combined.
3. Pour the mixture onto the baking sheet and spread into an even later.
4. Bake in the oven for 6 minutes. Remove the baking sheet from the oven and toss the mixture. Spread out into an even layer again and return the baking sheet to the oven; bake for another 6 minutes.
5. Remove baking sheet from the oven and let it cool for at least 5 minutes before enjoying.

● GENERAL DIET

Nutrition Facts (1/4 cup):
166 calories, 4g protein, 7.5g carbohydrates, 14.5g fat

TIPS/SUGGESTIONS:
- Add this granola to a low fat Greek yogurt or mix with a serving of berries for a yummy breakfast or snack.

Part Six: Lunch

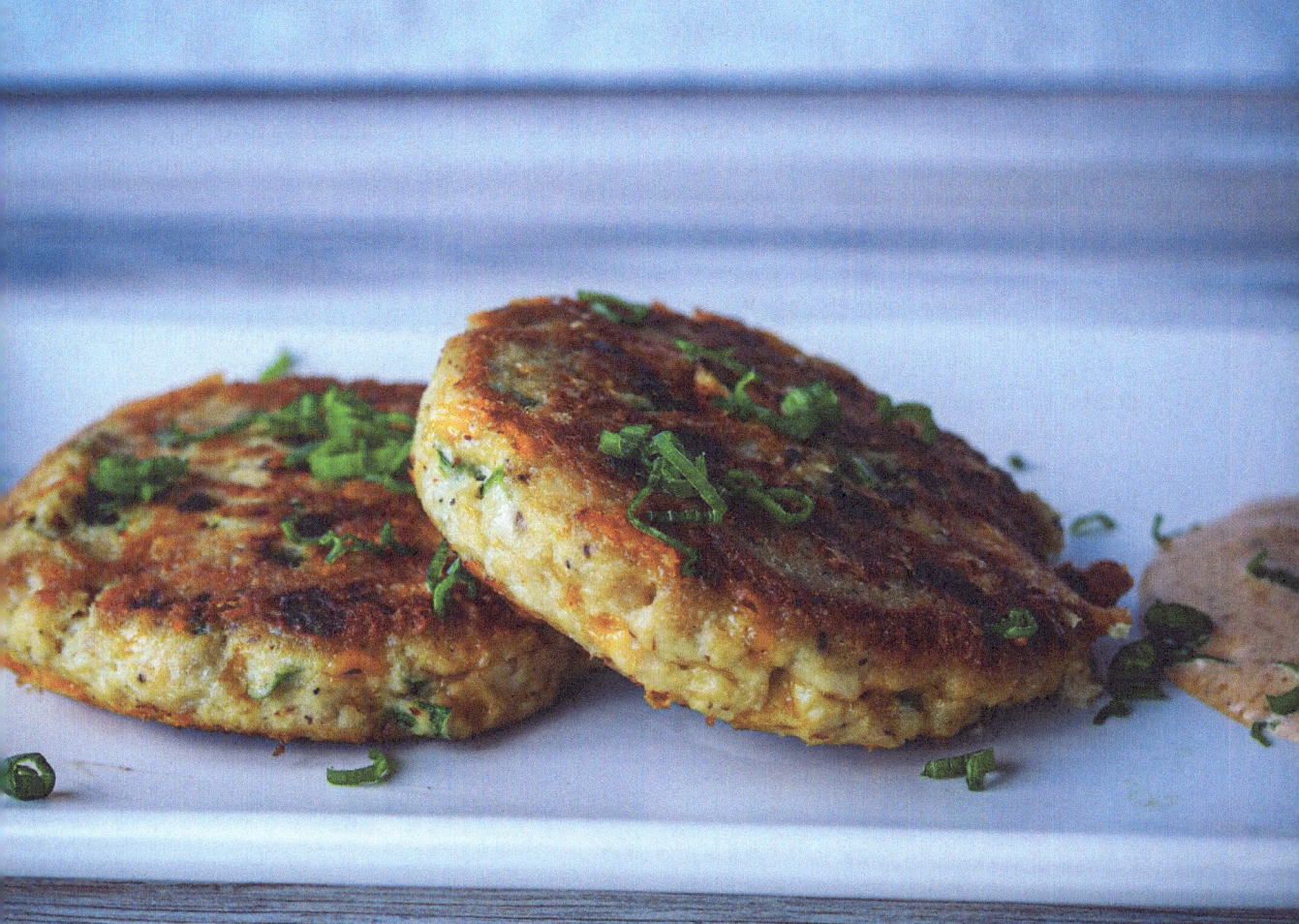

Part Six:
LUNCH

COBB SALAD

SERVINGS: 2 **MAKES: 1 1/2 CUPS** **TIME: 20 MINUTES**

INGREDIENTS:

1/4 cup romaine lettuce, chopped
1/4 cup spinach leaves, chopped
1-2 TBSP low calorie ranch dressing
2 ounces chicken, cooked and diced
2 slices turkey bacon, cooked and diced
1 hardboiled egg, chopped
1 TBSP blue cheese crumbles
2 TBSP cherry tomatoes, diced
2 TBSP avocado, diced
Pepper, to taste

DIRECTIONS:

1. Combine the romaine lettuce and spinach in a medium bowl. Add 1 TBSP ranch dressing and pepper to taste. Toss the leafy greens with the dressing until well coated.
2. Add the chicken, bacon, egg, blue cheese, tomatoes, and avocado to the bowl. Toss the ingredients together until well combined.
3. Add an additional 1 TBSP of ranch dressing and additional pepper if you would like and enjoy.

Nutrition Facts (1/2 of recipe):
174 calories, 12g protein, 2g carbohydrates, 12g fat

● **GENERAL DIET**
TIPS/SUGGESTIONS:
- Limit the dressing you use in salads by only dressing the part of a salad that needs flavor, like the leafy greens and vegetables.
- Experiment with herbs in your salad for extra flavor.
- Aim for ranch dressing that is 80 calories or less for 2 TBSP.

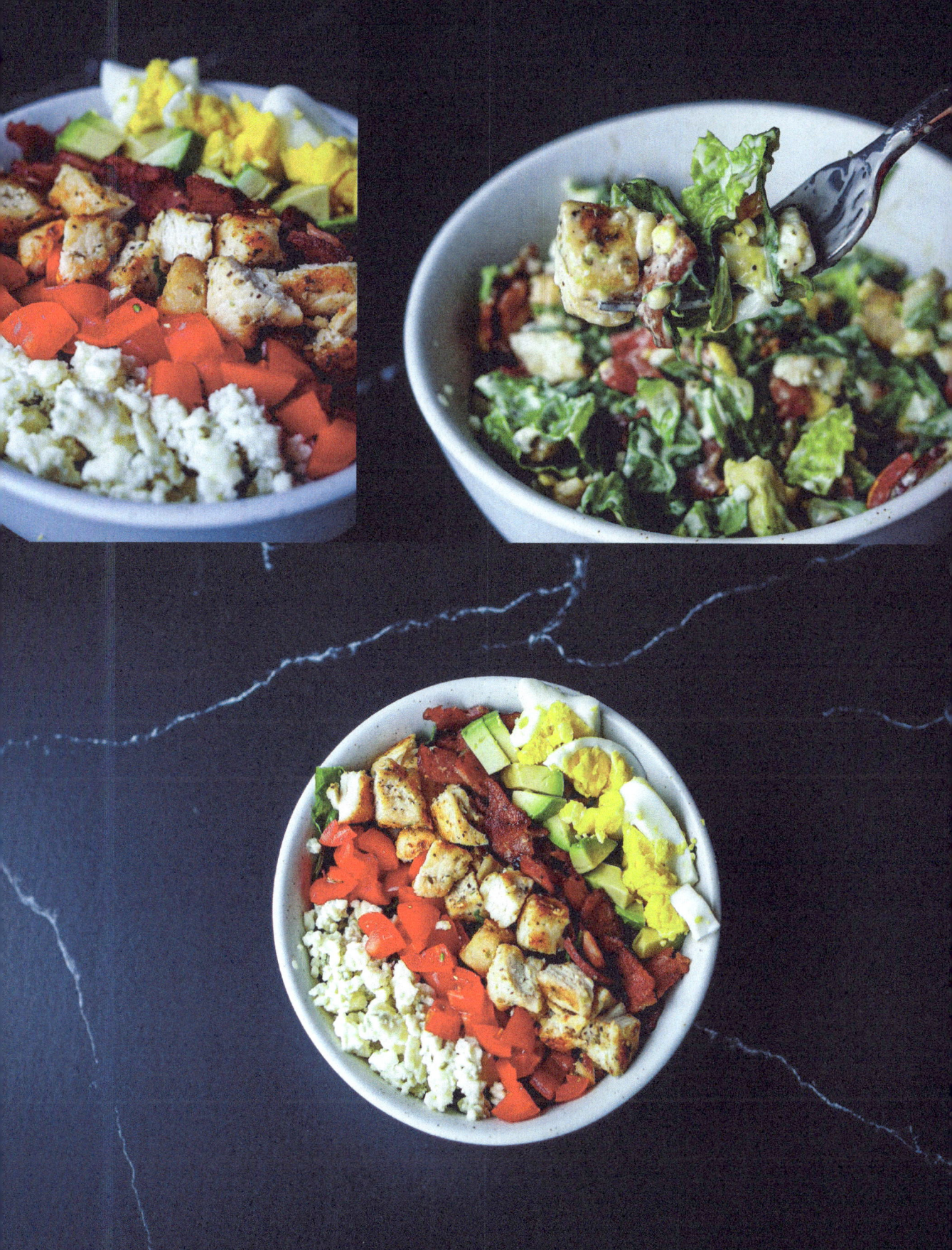

Part Six: Lunch

CHICKPEA TUNA SALAD

SERVINGS: 2-4   **MAKES: 1 1/2-2 CUPS**   **TIME: 15 MINUTES**

INGREDIENTS:

1 can tuna, canned in water and drained
1 TBSP light mayonnaise
1 TBSP hummus, plain
1 TBSP Dijon mustard
1/4 tsp salt
1/4 tsp pepper
1/4 tsp garlic powder
1/2 tsp dried dill
1/2 cup canned garbanzo beans, drained and rinsed
1/4 cup jicama, peeled and diced
1/4 cup cucumber, diced
2 TBSP feta cheese, crumbled

Optional topping:
Lemon Juice

DIRECTIONS:

1. Drain can of tuna and transfer to a medium sized bowl.
2. Add mayonnaise, hummus, Dijon mustard, salt, pepper, garlic powder, and dried dill to the bowl and mix until well combined with the tuna.
3. Add garbanzo beans (also known as chickpeas), jicama, cucumber, and feta cheese to the bowl.
4. Mix until well combined and drizzle with a little lemon juice if you desire!
5. You can eat this tuna salad as is; put it in a low carbohydrate tortilla or in a lettuce wrap for something different. This makes two to four servings depending on your portion sizes.

● **GENERAL DIET**

Nutrition Facts (3/4 cup):
160 calories, 14g protein, 13g carbohydrates, 7g fat

TIPS/SUGGESTIONS:
- This is a great recipe for making ahead of time and include for lunch during the week.
- Have you never used jicama? It's a great root vegetable to use in salads or as veggie sticks. Simply peel and chop.

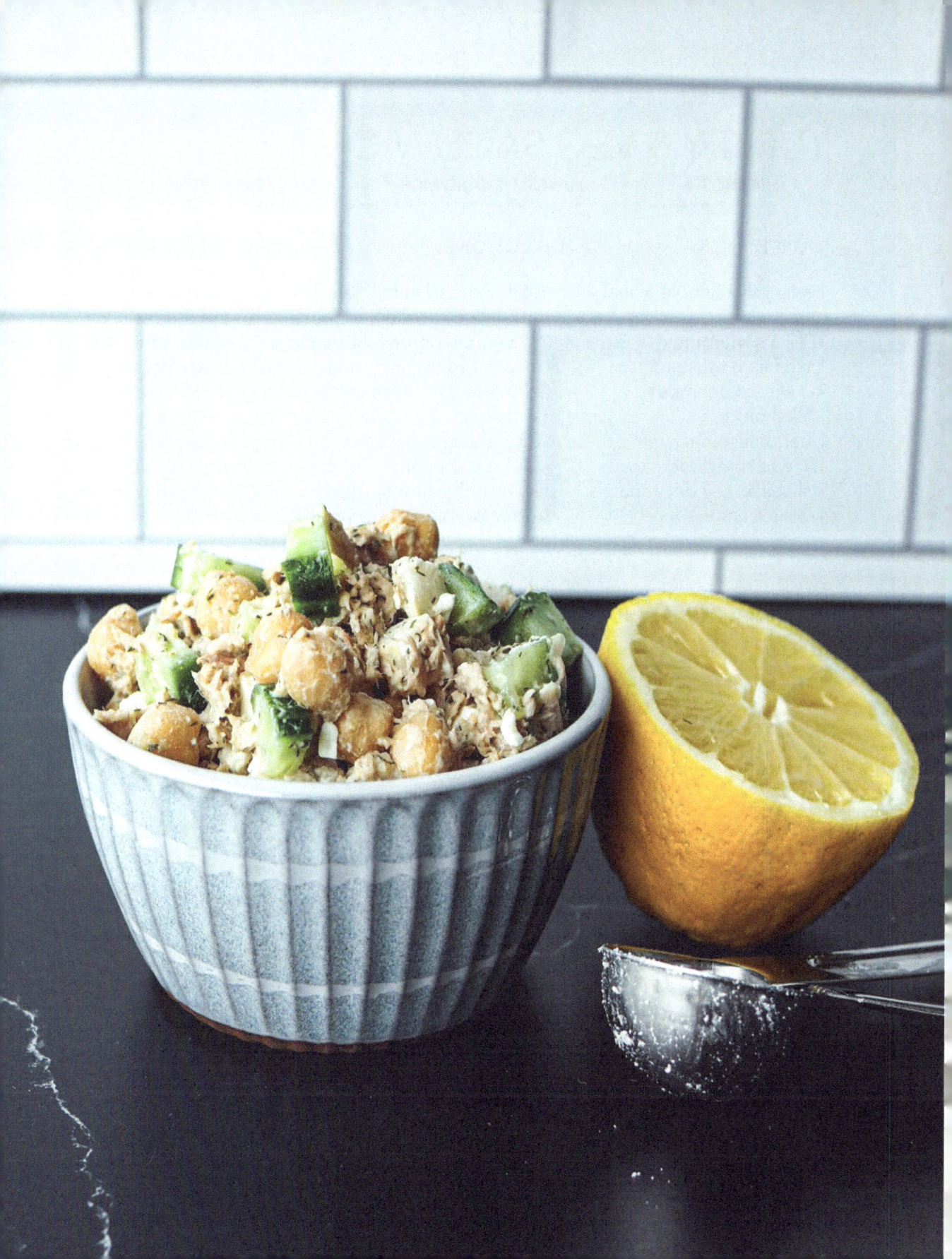

Part Six: Lunch

TURKEY & VEG SANDWICH

SERVINGS: 1 **MAKES: 1/2 SANDWICH** **TIME: 10 MINUTES**

INGREDIENTS:

1 small slice whole wheat bread
1/2 TBSP hummus
1 tsp Dijon mustard
2-3 slices cucumber
1 slice pickle
1 handful spinach leaves
1/4 cup shredded carrots
2 slices turkey deli meat
1/2 slice cheese

● GENERAL DIET

DIRECTIONS:

1. Slice bread in half lengthwise; spread hummus on one slice of bread and mustard on the other slice.
2. Layer cucumber slices, pickle, spinach, shredded carrots, turkey, and cheese on one slice of bread.
3. Put the two pieces of bread together to make your sandwich; cut in half and serve with a serving of fruit or vegetables.
4. A lot of patients are unable to tolerate bread until a few months after surgery. Keep this in mind when introducing bread into your diet and monitor your tolerance.

Nutrition Facts:
182 calories, 17g protein, 17g carbohydrates, 5.5g fat

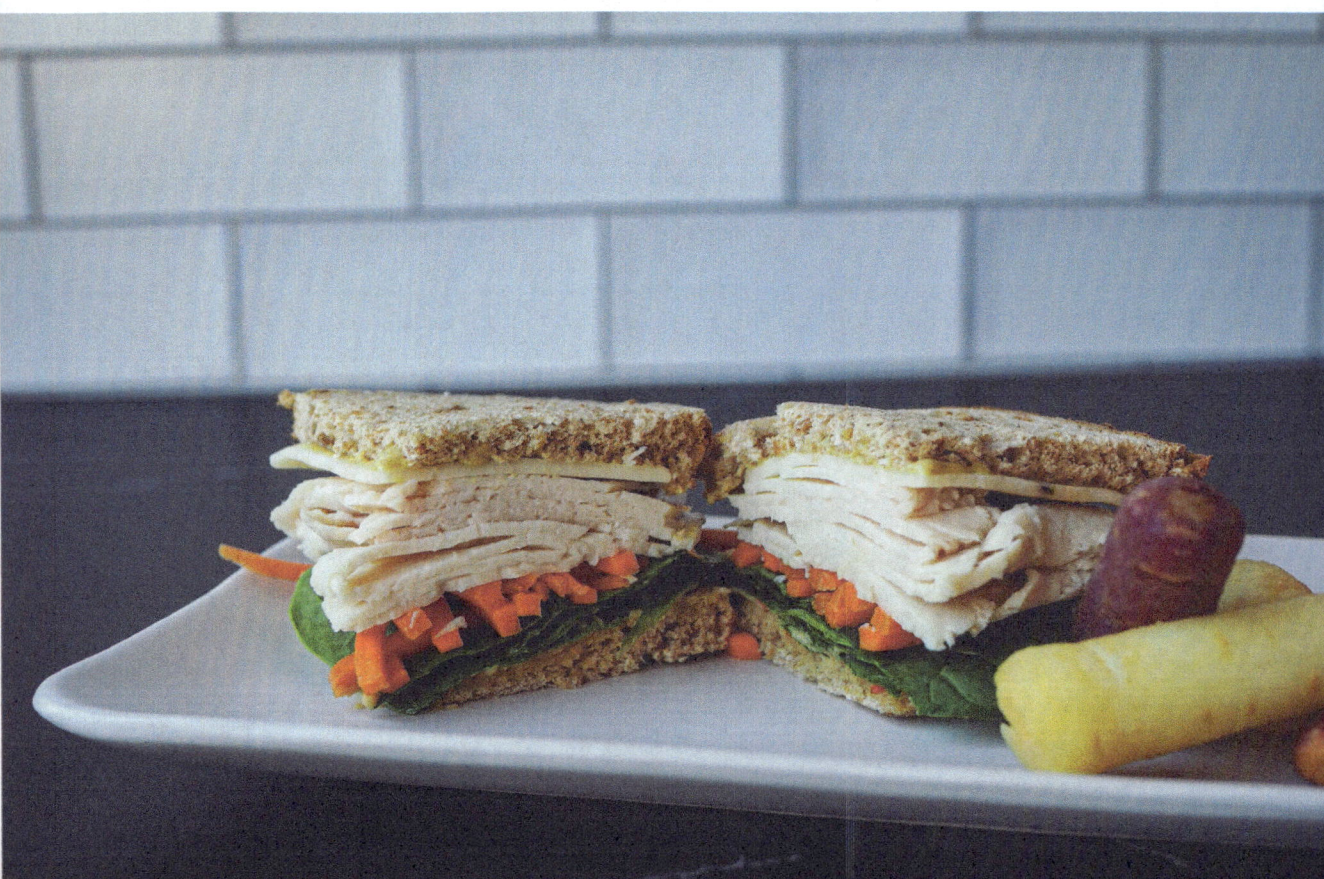

SESAME SALMON WRAP

SERVINGS: 1 **MAKES:** 1 WRAP **TIME:** 20 MINUTES

INGREDIENTS:

1 small low carbohydrate tortilla
1 TBSP hummus
1/4 cup fresh spinach, packed
2 TBSP shredded carrots
2 TBSP cucumber, diced
2 TBSP red bell pepper, diced
2 TBSP frozen edamame, shelled
1 2.5 ounce packet salmon
1 tsp sesame seeds

Marinade/sauce:
1 tsp sesame oil
1 1/2 TBSP low sodium soy sauce
2 tsp rice vinegar
1/8 tsp garlic powder
1/4 tsp fresh ginger, minced
1/8 tsp red pepper flakes
Salt to taste

DIRECTIONS:

1. Prepare the wrap by spreading hummus onto the low carbohydrate tortilla, then layer with spinach, carrots, cucumber, bell pepper, and edamame. Set aside.
2. In a small bowl, combine sesame oil, soy sauce, rice vinegar, garlic powder, ginger, red pepper flakes, and salt to taste.
3. Add salmon and sesame seeds to the same bowl and mix until the salmon is well-coated in the sauce.
4. Add the salmon mixture to the tortilla and roll up to enjoy.

● GENERAL DIET

Nutrition Facts:
287 calories, 25.5g protein, 27g carbohydrates, 14g fat

Part Six: Lunch

SAUSAGE AND POTATO SOUP

SERVINGS: 4-6 **MAKES:** ABOUT 4-5 CUPS **TIME:** 45 MINUTES

INGREDIENTS:

1/2 pound ground chicken sausage
1/2 cup yellow onion, diced
1 cup cauliflower florets, chopped
4 cloves garlic, minced
3 cups chicken broth
2 cups water
1 cup red potatoes, chopped
1 cup kale leaves, stemmed and chopped
3/4 tsp salt
3/4 tsp pepper
1 tsp dried thyme
1/2 tsp dried rosemary
1/4 cup half-and-half

DIRECTIONS:

1. Preheat a large pot over medium-high heat on the stove top.
2. Cook the ground chicken in the pot until browned and cooked through.
3. Add the onion, cauliflower florets, and garlic to the pot, cook for 3-4 minutes while stirring.
4. Add the chicken broth, water, red potatoes, and kale to the pot. While stirring occasionally bring to a boil and cover. Reduce heat to low, simmer for 15 minutes.
5. Add the salt, pepper, thyme, and rosemary. Cover again and simmer for another 5 minutes.
6. Remove the pot from heat, uncover, and let it cool for 10 minutes.
7. While continuously stirring the soup, slowly add in the half-and-half, stir well and you're done!

● GENERAL DIET

Nutrition Facts (1/4 of recipe, about 1 cup):
134 calories, 13.5g protein, 11g carbohydrates, 3.5g fat

TIPS/SUGGESTIONS:
- If you are unable to tolerate tough greens like kale you can try cooking it until it is very soft, substitute with spinach instead or simply don't add this ingredient to the recipe.

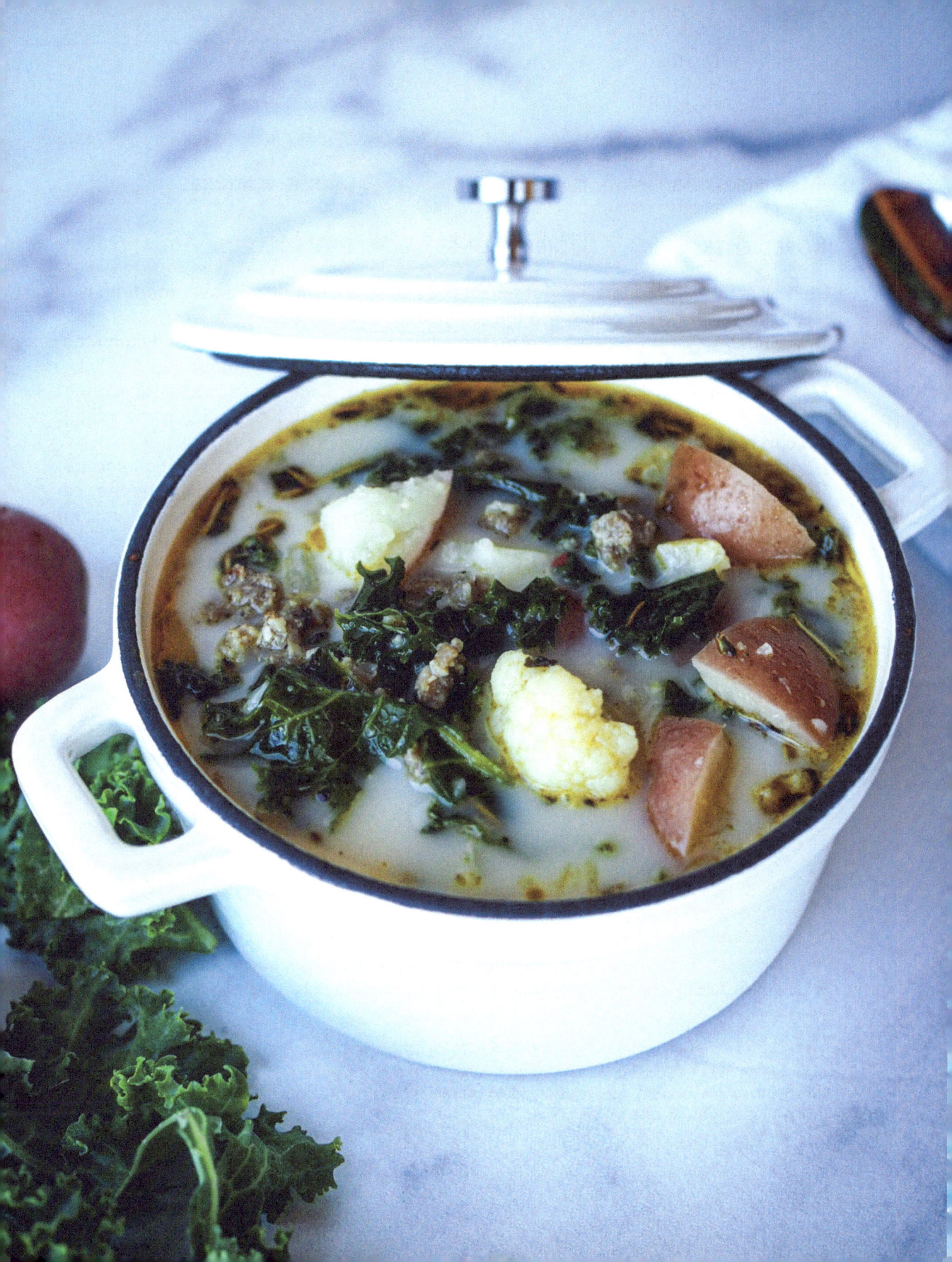

Part Six: Lunch

FIESTA CAULIFLOWER RICE

SERVINGS: 2-3   **MAKES: 2-3 CUPS**   **TIME: 25 MINUTES**

INGREDIENTS:

1 tsp olive oil
1 10oz package frozen cauliflower rice
1/4 cup frozen corn
1/4 cup canned black beans, rinsed and drained
1/3 cup salsa
1/2 tsp cumin
1 tsp chili powder
3-4 cloves garlic, minced
Salt and pepper, to taste

Optional ingredients:
4-8 ounces protein (chicken, steak, etc), fully cooked and diced
2 TBSP green onion, diced

DIRECTIONS:

1. Preheat olive oil in a medium pan over medium heat on the stove top.
2. Add the cauliflower rice and stir frequently until the rice begins to soften, about 6-8 minutes.
3. Add the frozen corn, black beans, and salsa. Continue to stir and allow the mixture to cook for an additional 3-4 minutes.
4. Add the cumin, chili powder and garlic. Salt and pepper the mixture to taste and cover. Cook while the pan is covered for about 5-6 minutes while the flavors come together.
5. Uncover the pan and cook until any liquid is evaporated while stirring the mixture occasionally.
6. Remove the pan from the heat and allow to cool for 2 minutes. Top with some green onion and your favorite protein option, and you have a great lunch!

● GENERAL DIET

Nutrition Facts (1/2 of recipe, about 1 cup):
105 calories, 5g protein, 21g carbohydrates, 0g fat

TIPS/SUGGESTIONS:
- Make sure to add your protein source for a balanced meal and adjust the nutrition facts as needed.
- You can use this recipe as meal when adding protein, or you can utilize it as is for a side dish on taco night.

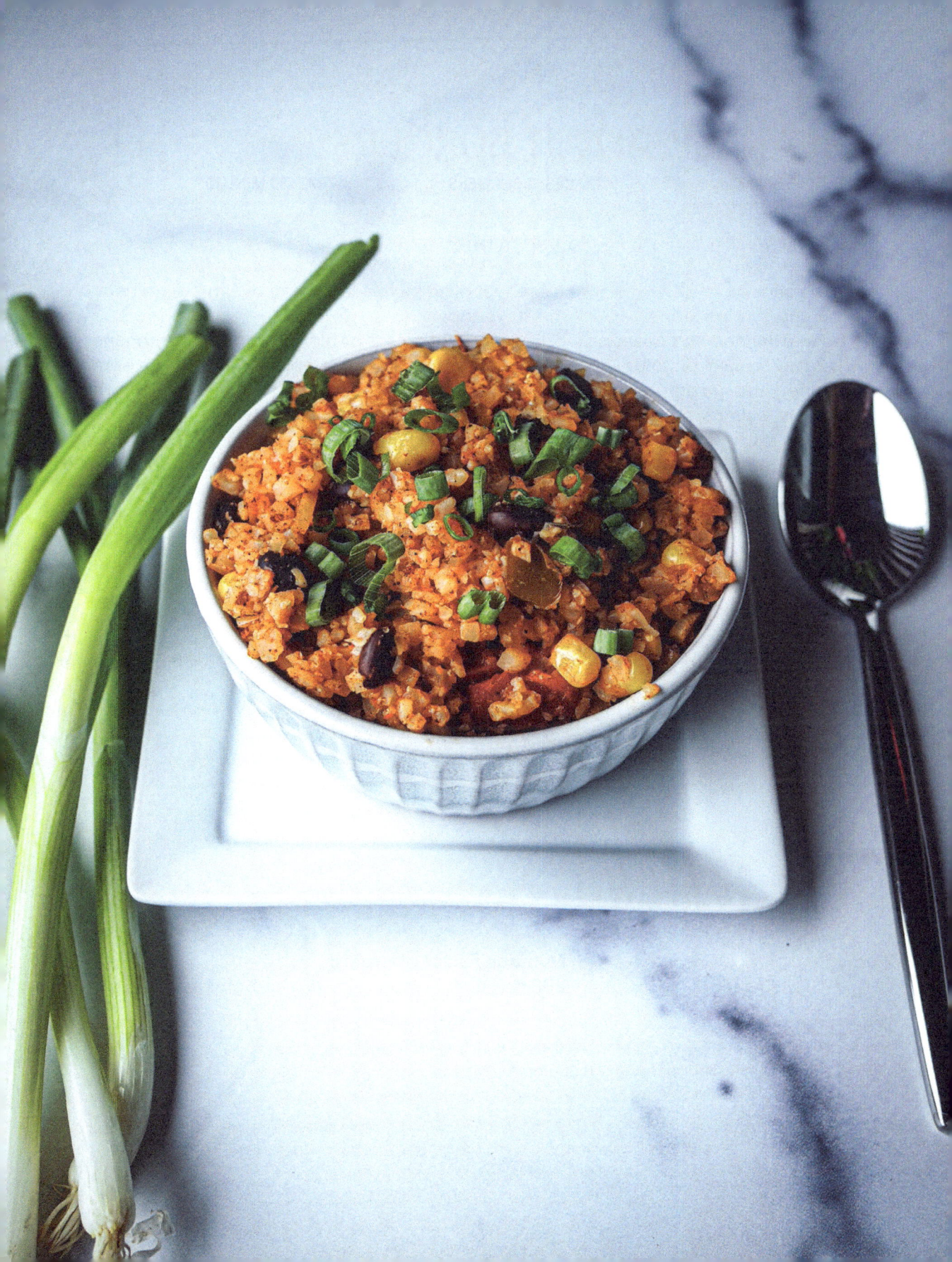

BEAN & WALNUT BURGERS

SERVINGS: 3   **MAKES: 3 BURGERS**   **TIME: 30 MINUTES**

INGREDIENTS:

1 tsp olive oil
1/2 cup canned kidney beans, drained and rinsed
1/2 cup canned pinto beans, drained and rinsed
1/4 cup walnuts, chopped
1/4 tsp salt
1/4 tsp pepper
2-3 garlic cloves, minced
1 TBSP fresh rosemary, minced
1 egg
1 TBSP almond flour
1 TBSP red onion, diced
2 TBSP Parmesan cheese (optional)
1 1/2 cups fresh spinach, packed
3 TBSP Italian salad dressing

DIRECTIONS:

1. Preheat olive oil in a large pan over medium heat on the stove top.
2. In a food processor or blender, add kidney beans, pinto beans, walnuts, salt, pepper, garlic, and rosemary. Blend together until well combined, then transfer the mixture to a medium-sized bowl.
3. Add the egg, almond flour, red onion, and Parmesan cheese. Using a wooden spoon or clean hands, mix the ingredients together.
4. Measure out approximately 1/4 cup of the mixture and roll into a ball using your hands. Flatten each ball to create a burger and place onto the hot pan.
5. Cook each burger on both sides for about 5-6 minutes or until each side is brown and crisp.
6. In a small bowl, toss together 1/2 cup of spinach with 1 TBSP of Italian salad dressing. Serve each burger over the lettuce and enjoy!

● **GENERAL DIET**

Nutrition Facts (1 burger):
208 calories, 11g protein, 19g carbohydrates, 11g fat

TIPS/SUGGESTIONS:
- If your mixture is too wet, add more almond flour 1 tsp at a time until you have the desired consistency for burgers.

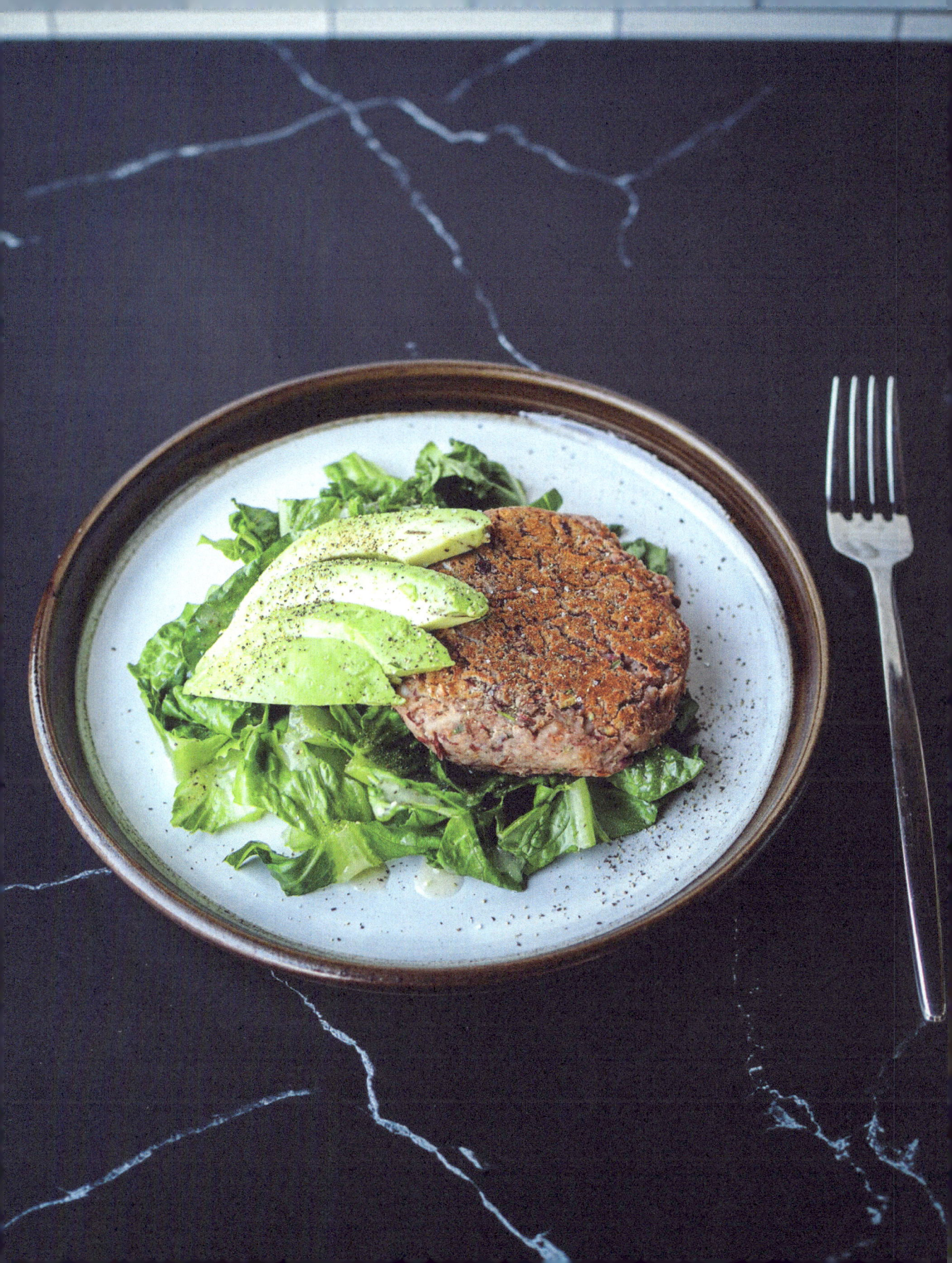

Part Six: Lunch

CHICKEN GRAPE & WALNUT SALAD

SERVINGS: 4 **MAKES: 2 CUPS** **TIME: 20 MINUTES**

INGREDIENTS:

1 cup chicken, cooked and shredded
1/4 cup light mayonnaise
1 TBSP Dijon mustard
1/2 tsp salt
1/2 tsp pepper
1/4 cup celery, diced
1/4 cup crushed walnuts
1/2 cup grapes, sliced in half
2 TBSP red onion, diced
1 TBSP tarragon, minced

Optional:
Lettuce for lettuce wrap (I like using romaine, but you can use green leaf or butter leaf as well)

DIRECTIONS:

1. Add chicken, mayonnaise, Dijon mustard, salt and pepper to a medium bowl. Stir until well combined and the chicken is evenly coated with the dressing.
2. Add celery, walnuts, grapes, red onion and tarragon to the bowl. Stir well and serve!

● **GENERAL DIET**

Nutrition Facts (1/2 cup):
165 calories, 11g protein, 4g carbohydrates, 14g fat

TIPS/SUGGESTIONS:
- You can eat this chicken salad in a lettuce wrap or in a low carbohydrate tortilla (as tolerated).

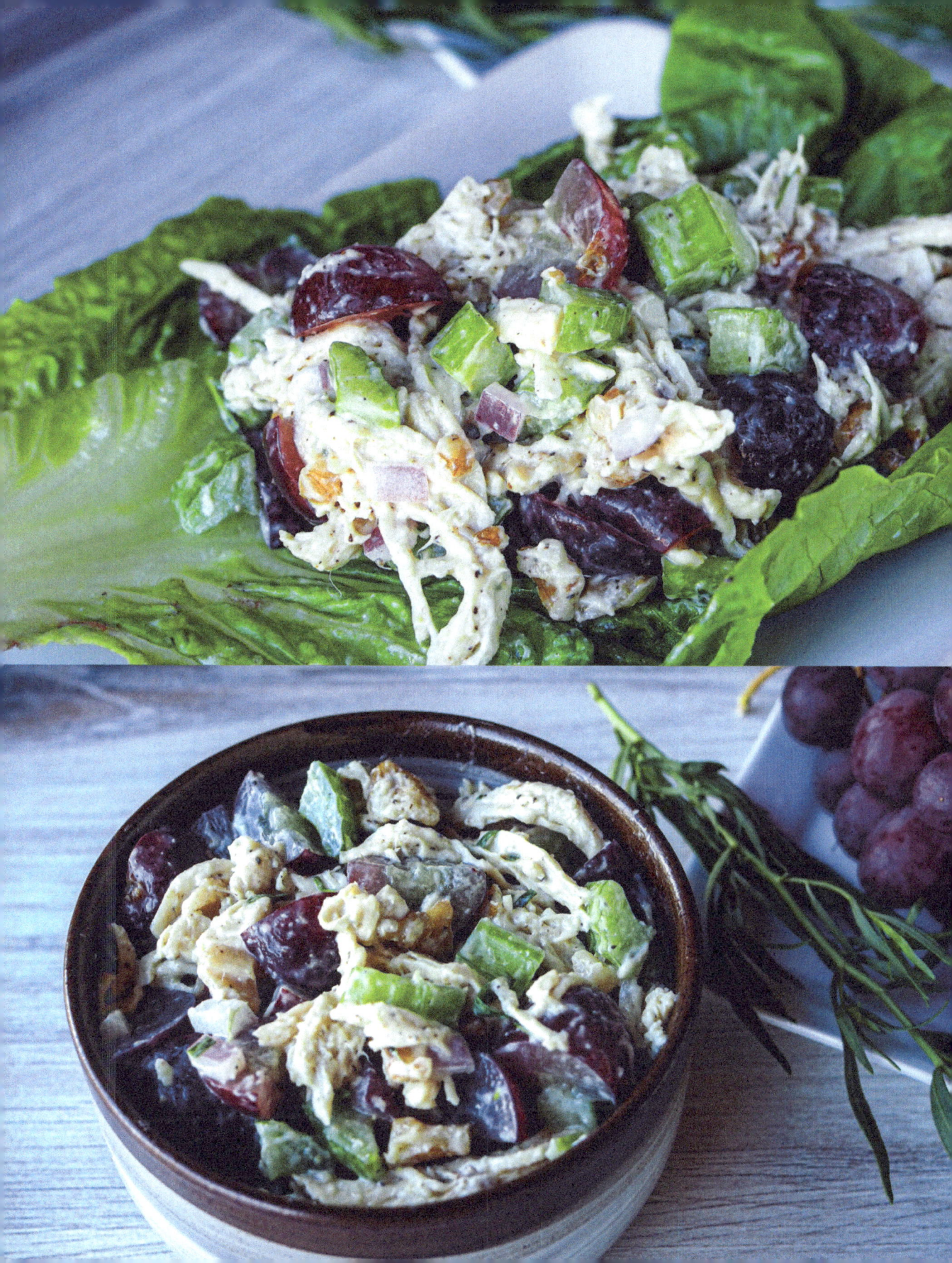

CHICKPEA BURGER WITH CAESAR SALAD

SERVINGS: 5   **MAKES:** 5 BURGERS   **TIME:** 25 MINUTES

INGREDIENTS:

2 tsp olive oil
1 can garbanzo beans (chickpeas), drained and rinsed
1/4 cup shredded Parmesan cheese
2 TBSP pine nuts
1/2 tsp salt
1/2 tsp pepper
1/4 tsp paprika
1/4 tsp dried oregano
1/2 tsp dried parsley
1 egg
2 TBSP almond flour
3-4 cloves garlic, minced
2-3 cups romaine lettuce, chopped
5 TBSP low calorie caesar dressing
5 TBSP Parmesan cheese
Pepper, to taste

DIRECTIONS:

1. Preheat olive oil in a large pan over medium heat on the stove top.
2. In a small food processor add the garbanzo beans, 1/4 cup Parmesan cheese, pine nuts, salt, pepper, paprika, oregano, parsley, egg, almond flour and garlic. Process/blend together until a smooth consistency (it's okay if there are some chunks of beans or cheese).
3. Measure out 2.5 ounces of the bean mixture and using your hands, roll into a ball then flatten into a burger. This recipe makes about five 2.5 ounce burgers.
4. Place each burger onto the hot pan and allow to cook on each side until brown and crisp, about 4-5 minutes per side.
5. While the burgers are cooking, combine 1/4-1/2 cup romaine lettuce and 1 TBSP of caesar dressing in a small bowl and toss to combine.
6. Top the salad with 1 TBSP Parmesan cheese, pepper to taste and 1 burger and you are set.

● GENERAL DIET

Nutrition Facts (as portioned in step #6):
223 calories, 11.5g protein, 17g carbohydrates, 12.5g fat

BEAN AND VEGETABLE SOUP

SERVINGS: 4   **MAKES: ABOUT 4 CUPS**   **TIME: 40 MINUTES**

INGREDIENTS:

1 tsp olive oil
1/4 cup onion, diced
1/4 cup celery, diced
1/2 cup asparagus, diced
2-3 cloves garlic, minced
1 large handful of spinach leaves
1 tsp salt
1/2 tsp pepper
1/2 tsp Italian seasoning
1 TBSP basil pesto
1/2 cup canned kidney beans, drained and rinsed
1/2 cup canned cannellini beans, drained and rinsed
2-3 cups vegetable broth
1/4 cup quinoa

DIRECTIONS:

1. Preheat olive oil in a large pot over medium-high heat on the stove top.
2. Add the onion, celery, asparagus, and garlic to the pot. Stir until the vegetables are well coated in the oil. While continuing to stir occasionally, allow the vegetables to cook until they begin to soften, about 4-5 minutes.
3. Add the spinach to the pot and stir until the spinach is wilted.
4. Add the salt, pepper, Italian seasoning, and pesto to the pot. Stir and allow to cook with the vegetables for 2-3 minutes.
5. Add the beans, broth and quinoa to the pot and bring the mixture to a boil. Cover and reduce the heat to low, simmer the soup for 15-20 minutes or until the vegetables are soft and the quinoa is cooked. Add additional broth if needed. If enjoying this recipe on a soft foods diet cook the vegetables and quinoa until very soft.

- SOFT FOODS DIET
- GENERAL DIET

Nutrition Facts (1 cup):
144 calories, 7g protein, 23g protein, 3g fat

Part Six: Lunch

JALAPENO CHEDDAR SALMON CAKES

SERVINGS: 2-4 **MAKES: 4-5 CAKES** **TIME: 25 MINUTES**

INGREDIENTS:

1 tsp olive oil
1/2 jalapeno, seeds removed and diced
3 cloves garlic, minced
2 TBSP green onion, diced
5 ounces canned salmon
1/4 cup shredded cheddar cheese
1/4 tsp salt
1/4 tsp pepper
1 egg
1/2 TBSP almond flour
1/8 tsp paprika

DIRECTIONS:

1. Preheat olive oil in a medium pan over medium heat on the stove top.
2. Cook the jalapeno, garlic, and green onion in the preheated pan until fragrant and the jalapeno begins to soften, approximately 4-5 minutes. If using this recipe on a soft foods diet make sure to cook these ingredients until they are very soft.
3. Transfer this mixture to a small bowl or plate and allow to cool for 2-3 minutes.
4. Place the pan back onto the stove top on medium heat to keep it warm.
5. In a medium-sized bowl, combine salmon, cooled jalapeno mixture, shredded cheese, salt, pepper, egg, almond flour, and paprika. Stir until well combined.
6. Measure out about 2.5 ounces of salmon mixture and roll into a ball using your hands. Flatten each ball to create the salmon cakes and place each cake onto the heated pan.
7. Cook for about 3-4 minutes on each side or until slightly browned and crisp. Remove from the pan and enjoy!

- SOFT FOODS DIET
- GENERAL DIET

Nutrition Facts (1/4 of recipe, about 1 salmon cake):
90 calories, 9g protein, 0.5g carbohydrates, 5.5g fat

TIPS/SUGGESTIONS:
- Pair these salmon cakes with some well-roasted vegetables (soft foods diet) or a leafy green salad with a low calorie dressing (general diet).

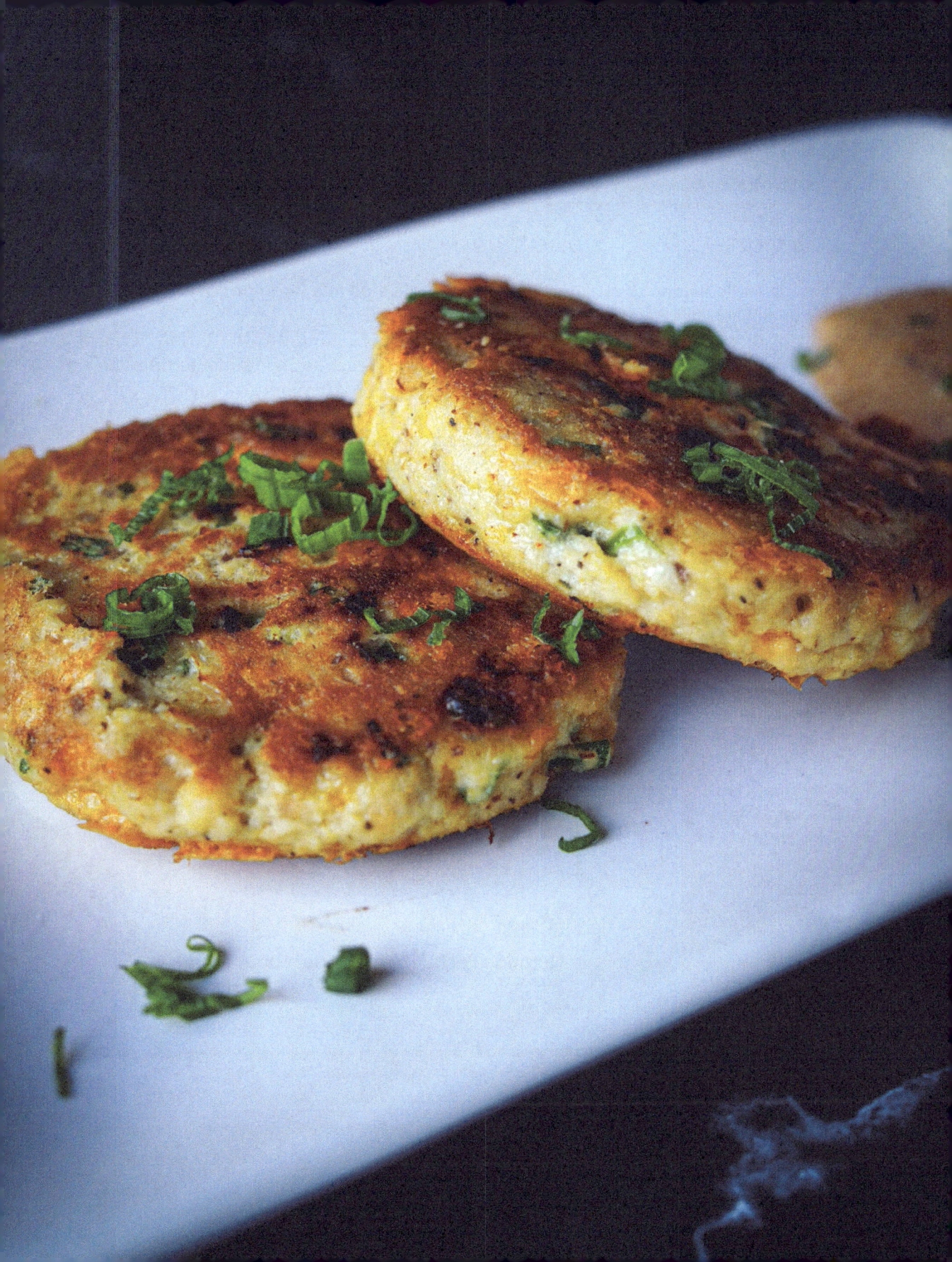

Part Six: Lunch

CHICKEN TORTILLA SOUP

SERVINGS: 4-5   **MAKES: 4-5 CUPS**   **TIME: 45 MINUTES**

INGREDIENTS:

2 tsp olive oil, divided
1 large chicken breast (10-12 ounces), diced
1/4 cup onion, diced
1/2 cup green bell pepper, diced
1/2 cup shredded carrots
1/2 jalapeno, seeds removed and diced
3-4 cloves garlic, minced
Juice of 1/2 lime
1 tsp salt
1 TBSP chili powder
1 tsp cumin
1 tsp oregano
1 14-ounce can of diced tomatoes
1 14-ounce can of black beans, drained and rinsed
2 cups chicken broth

Optional toppings:
Sour cream
Cheese
Avocado
Tortilla strips

DIRECTIONS:

1. Preheat 1 tsp olive oil in a large pot over medium heat on the stove top.
2. Add chicken to the pot and brown, stirring occasionally until the chicken reaches an internal temperature of 165 degrees F, about 8- 10 minutes. Transfer chicken to a small bowl or plate and set aside.
3. Preheat 1 tsp olive oil in a large pot over medium heat on the stove top.
4. Add onion, bell pepper, carrots, jalapeno, garlic, and lime juice to the pot and stir. Cook until the vegetables begin to soften, about 6 minutes while stirring occasionally.
5. Add salt, chili powder, cumin, and oregano to the vegetable mixture and stir until well combined.
6. Add diced tomatoes, black beans and chicken to the pot and stir well. Cook until the mixture comes to a boil, about 6-8 minutes.
7. Add the chicken broth to the pot and bring to a boil. Once the soup is boiling, cover and reduce heat to low. Simmer for about 10 minutes while stirring occasionally.
8. Remove pot from heat, uncover and allow to cool for 5 minutes before eating.

● **GENERAL DIET**

Nutrition Facts (1/4 of recipe, about 1 cup):
281 calories, 28g protein, 29g carbohydrates, 4.5g fat

TIPS/SUGGESTIONS:
- Nutrition facts do not include optional toppings.
- This recipe offers a high-protein content along with a high fiber content which will help you feel full and satisfied for hours.

GARDEN VEGETABLE CHAFFLE

SERVINGS: 2 **MAKES: 1 LARGE CHAFFLE** **TIME: 15 MINUTES**

INGREDIENTS:

1 tsp olive oil
2 TBSP shredded carrots
2 TBSP shredded zucchini
1 TBSP green onion, diced
1 egg
2 TBSP cream cheese, whipped
1/4 tsp baking powder
1 TBSP almond flour
1/4 tsp dried parsley
Salt/pepper, to taste

● GENERAL DIET

DIRECTIONS:

1. Preheat a small waffle iron. Preheat olive oil in a small pan over medium heat on the stove top.
3. Add carrots, zucchini, and onion to the pan. While stirring occasionally, let the vegetable mixture cook until the vegetables have softened, about 5-6 minutes. Remove the pan from the heat and set aside to cool.
5. Mix together the egg, cream cheese, baking powder, almond flour, parsley, salt, and pepper in a small bowl. Whisk together with a fork until well combined.
6. Mix in the vegetables and pour the mixture into the waffle iron and cook until lightly browned, about 2 minutes.

Nutrition Facts (1/2 chaffle):
113 calories, 4.5g protein, 2g carbohydrates, 9.5g fat

MEAT & VEGETABLE RICE CAKE

SERVINGS: 1 **MAKES: 1 RICE CAKE** **TIME: 8 MINUTES**

INGREDIENTS:

1 rice cake
2 TBSP cream cheese
2 TBSP sprouts
2-4 spinach leaves
2 slices deli meat
3-4 slices of cucumber
Salt/pepper, to taste

Optional toppings:
1/2 TBSP hot sauce

● GENERAL DIET

DIRECTIONS:

1. Spread cream cheese evenly over the rice cake.
2. Layer the rice cake with sprouts, spinach leaves, deli meat and cucumber.
3. Sprinkle with salt and pepper to taste and drizzle with hot sauce if you want to spice it up.

You can also use other vegetables you enjoy like bell pepper, shredded carrots, or even avocado or pickles. Also, consider using other herbs and spices to create the flavor you want.

Nutrition Facts:
153 calories, 12g protein, 9g carbohydrates, 7g fat

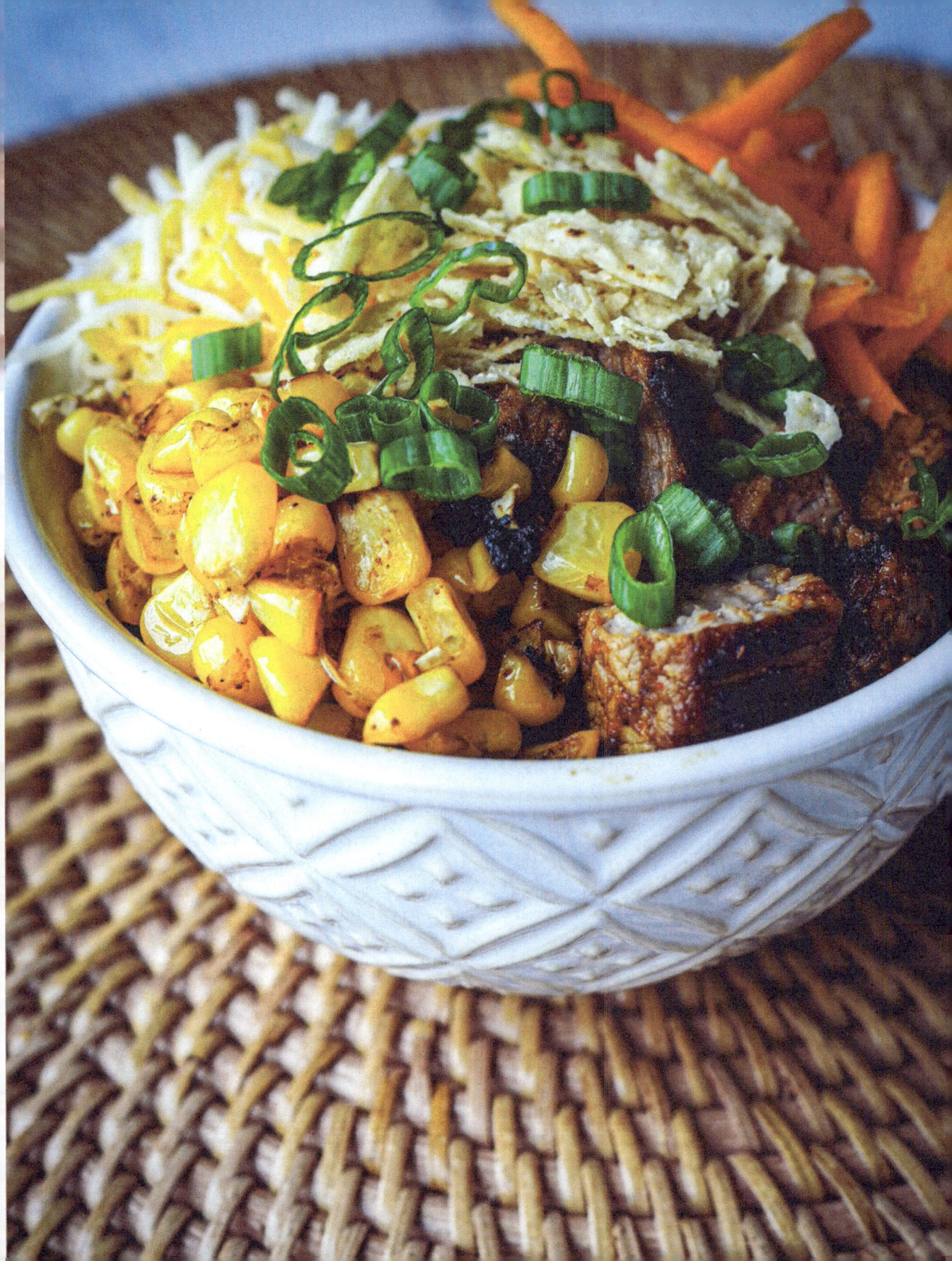

TACO SALAD

SERVINGS: 1 **MAKES: 1 CUP** **TIME: 30 MINUTES**

INGREDIENTS:

1 tsp olive oil
2 TBSP corn
2 ounces steak, diced
1 tsp chili powder
1/2 tsp cumin
1/4 cup romaine lettuce, chopped
1 TBSP shredded cheese
1 TBSP shredded carrots
1 TBSP tortilla chips
1/2 TBSP green onion
1 TBSP salsa
1 TBSP sour cream
Salt/pepper, to taste

DIRECTIONS:

1. Preheat olive oil in a small pan over medium heat on the stove top.
2. Add the corn and steak to the pan and season with chili powder, cumin, and a pinch of salt and pepper.
3. While stirring occasionally, allow the mixture to cook on the stove top until the steak is cooked through, about 8 minutes.
4. Transfer the corn and steak to a small plate and set aside to cool.
5. In a medium-sized bowl mix together lettuce, cheese, carrots, tortilla chips, and green onion. Set aside.
6. In a small bowl mix together the salsa and sour cream. Add the salsa mixture to the lettuce mixture and toss until fully coated.
7. Add the corn and steak to the salad and toss together until well combined.

● GENERAL DIET

Nutrition Facts:
281 calories, 14g protein, 11g carbohydrates, 18g fat

TIPS/SUGGESTIONS:
- If you struggle with tolerating leafy greens, you can choose to not include the romaine lettuce and still have a great meal.
- Remind yourself to chew foods thoroughly before swallowing especially with raw vegetables.

Part Six: Lunch

ASPARAGUS PESTO CHAFFLE

SERVINGS: 2 **MAKES:** 1 LARGE CHAFFLE **TIME:** 15 MINUTES

INGREDIENTS:

1 TBSP basil pesto
1/4 cup asparagus, chopped
Salt/pepper, to taste
1 egg
1/4 cup shredded Parmesan cheese
1/4 tsp baking powder
1 TBSP almond flour

● GENERAL DIET

DIRECTIONS:

1. Preheat a small waffle iron.
2. Preheat small pan over medium heat on the stove top. Add asparagus and pesto; stir frequently until asparagus begins to soften, about 5 minutes. Remove from heat and set aside to cool.
3. Combine egg, Parmesan cheese, baking powder, almond flour, and asparagus mixture in a small bowl. Whisk to combine; add salt and pepper to taste.
4. Pour mixture into the waffle iron and cook until lightly browned, about 2 minutes.
5. Top with sour cream and sprinkle of Parmesan cheese.

Nutrition Facts (1/2 chaffle):
131 calories, 8g protein, 3g carbohydrates, 9g fat

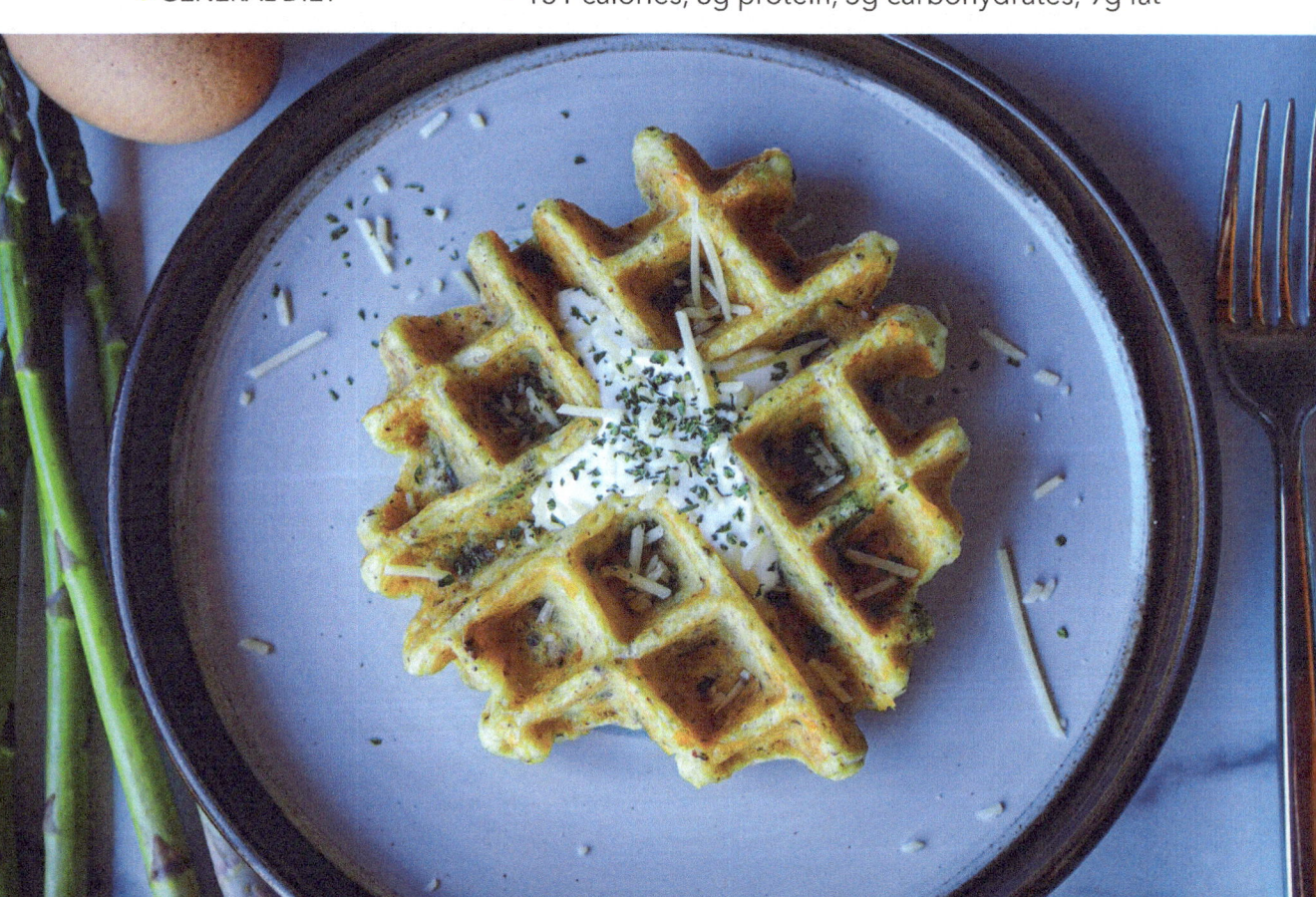

BUFFALO CHICKEN CHAFFLE

SERVINGS: 2   **MAKES:** 1 LARGE CHAFFLE   **TIME:** 20 MINUTES

INGREDIENTS:

3 ounces ground chicken, fully cooked and cooled
1 TBSP buffalo hot sauce
1 egg
1/4 cup shredded mozzarella cheese
1 TBSP almond flour
1/4 tsp baking powder
1/4 tsp garlic powder
Salt/pepper, to taste

Optional ingredient:
Low calorie ranch dressing
● GENERAL DIET

DIRECTIONS:

1. Preheat a small waffle iron.
2. Combine cooked chicken and buffalo sauce in a small bowl.
3. Add egg, cheese, almond flour, baking powder, garlic powder, salt, and pepper to the bowl. Whisk with a fork until well combined.
4. Pour mixture into the waffle iron and cook until lightly browned, about 2 minutes.
5. Top with additional buffalo hot sauce and use low calorie ranch dressing as a dipping sauce if you would like.

Nutrition Facts (1/2 chaffle):
151 calories, 17g protein, 2g carbohydrates, 8g fat

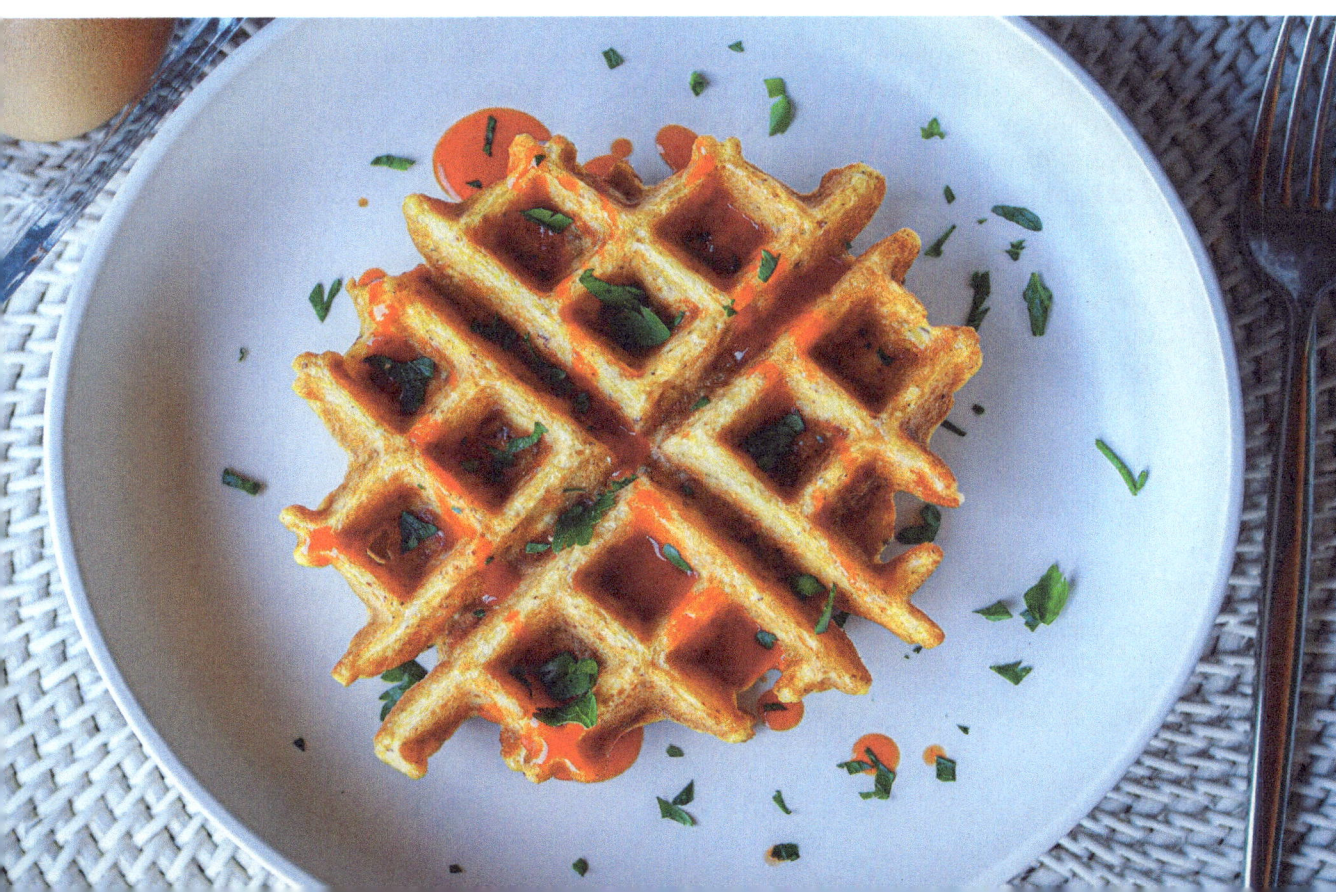

Part Six: Lunch
BEEF & BEAN JALAPENO CHILI

SERVINGS: 7 **MAKES: ABOUT 7 CUPS** **TIME: 40 MINUTES**

INGREDIENTS:

1 TBSP oil
1 pound lean ground beef
1/2 onion, peeled and diced
1 green bell pepper, diced
1 jalapeno, seeds removed and diced
1 TBSP tomato paste
1 14-ounce can diced tomatoes
1 cup canned pinto beans, drained and rinsed
1 cup canned kidney beans, drained and rinsed
1 tsp salt
1/2 tsp pepper
3-4 cloves garlic, minced
1 1/2 TBSP chili powder
1/2 tsp thyme
1/2 tsp paprika
32oz beef broth

Optional toppings:
Avocado
Sour Cream
Cheese

DIRECTIONS:

1. Add the oil to a large pot and place it over medium-high heat on the stove top. Once the oil is hot, add the ground beef and use a wooden spoon to break it up. Cook for 6-8 minutes or until browned, stirring occasionally.
2. Add onion, bell pepper, and jalapeno to the pot. Cook until the vegetables begin to soften, about 5-6 minutes, stirring occasionally.
3. Once the beef is browned and the vegetables are beginning to soften, add tomato paste and stir to coat the beef and vegetables. Cook for 1-2 minutes.
4. Add the entire can of diced tomatoes (juices included), pinto beans, and kidney beans to the pot. Stir well.
5. Add salt, pepper, garlic, chili powder, thyme, and paprika to the pot and stir to combine.
6. Pour beef broth in the pot and bring to a boil. Once the pot is boiling, cover and reduce heat to low. Simmer while covered for about 20 minutes, stirring occasionally.
7. Remove pot from the heat and allow to cool for 5 minutes before eating.
8. Add optional toppings as desired and enjoy!

● **GENERAL DIET**

Nutrition Facts (1 cup):
229 calories, 19g protein, 18g carbohydrates, 9g fat

TIPS/SUGGESTIONS:
- This recipe is great for batch cooking and also a great recipe for the entire family.
- The nutrition facts above do not include optional toppings

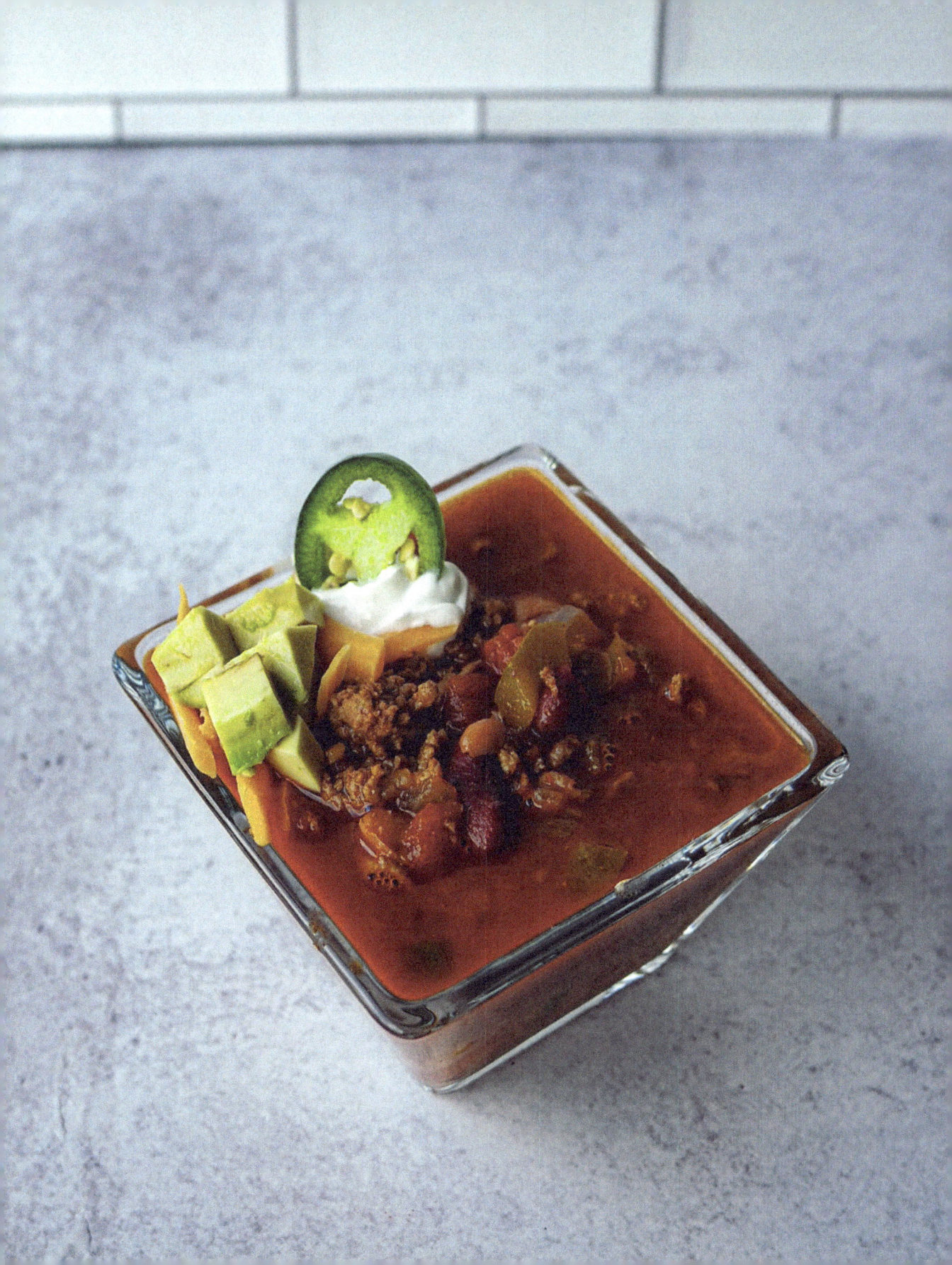

APPLE PECAN SALAD

SERVINGS: 1 **MAKES:** 3/4 CUP **TIME:** 10 MINUTES

INGREDIENTS:

Salad:
1/2 cup romaine lettuce, chopped
1 TBSP feta cheese
1 TBSP red onion, diced
1 TBSP pecans, chopped
1 TBSP green apple, diced

Dressing:
1/2 TBSP olive oil
1 TBSP balsamic vinegar
1/2 tsp Dijon mustard
1/8 tsp garlic powder
Pinch of salt and pepper

Optional ingredient:
2-3 ounces lean steak, diced and fully cooked

DIRECTIONS:

1. In a small bowl add the lettuce, feta cheese, red onion, pecans, and green apple; toss until combined.
2. In a separate small bowl, combine olive oil, balsamic vinegar, mustard, garlic powder, salt, and pepper. Whisk ingredients with a fork until well combined.
3. Pour the salad dressing over the lettuce mixture and toss the ingredients until everything is coated in the dressing.
4. You can use this recipe as a side to whatever you are cooking or add a portion of protein to make it a meal on it's own.

● **GENERAL DIET**

Nutrition Facts (1 salad + 2 ounces lean steak):
296 calories, 16.5g protein, 7g carbohydrates, 22g fat

TIPS/SUGGESTIONS:
- If you want to make this salad ahead of time, store the salad dressing separate from the salad in an airtight container and in the refrigerator. Add the salad dressing when you are ready to eat.

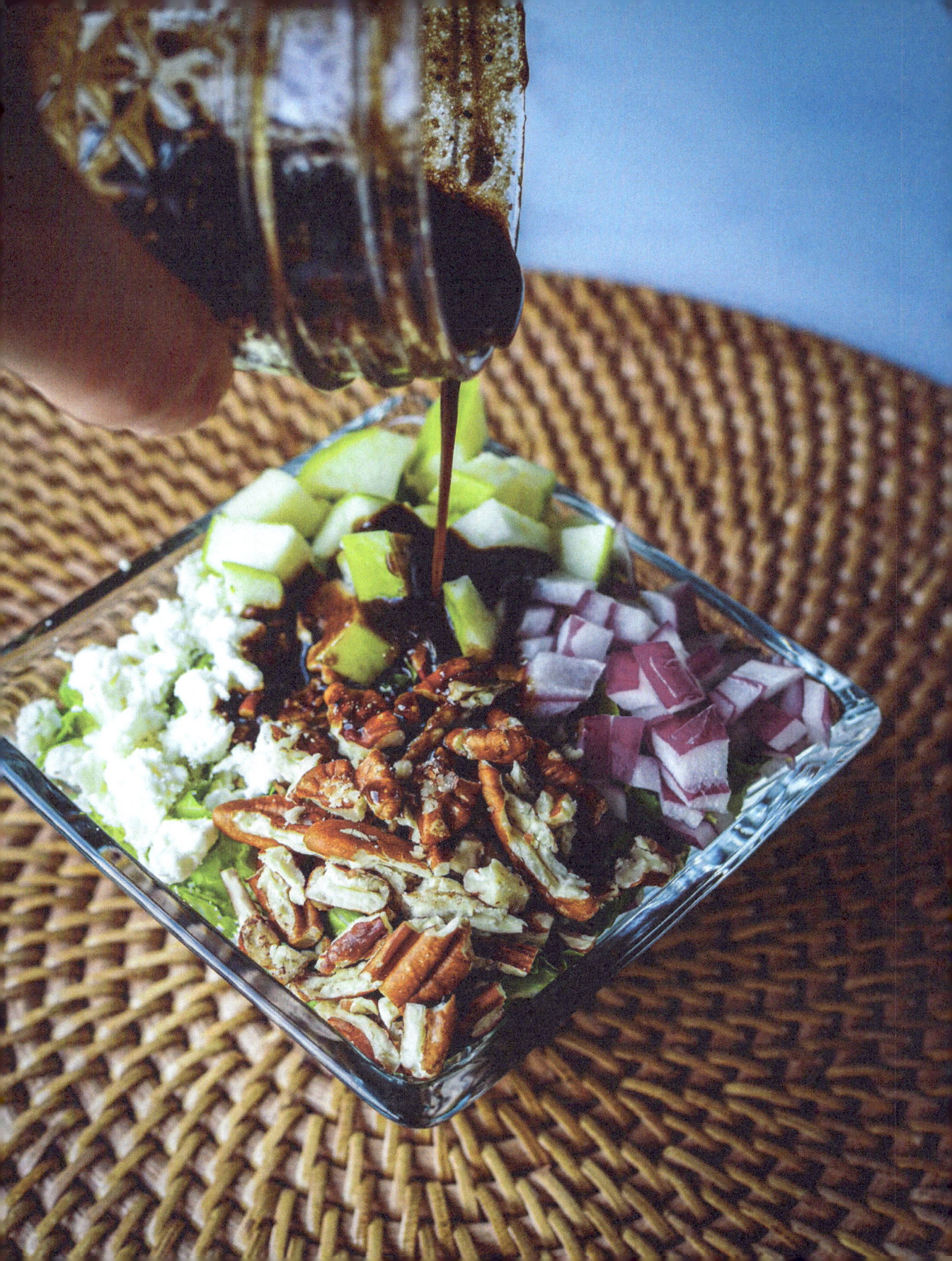

# Part Seven: Dinner

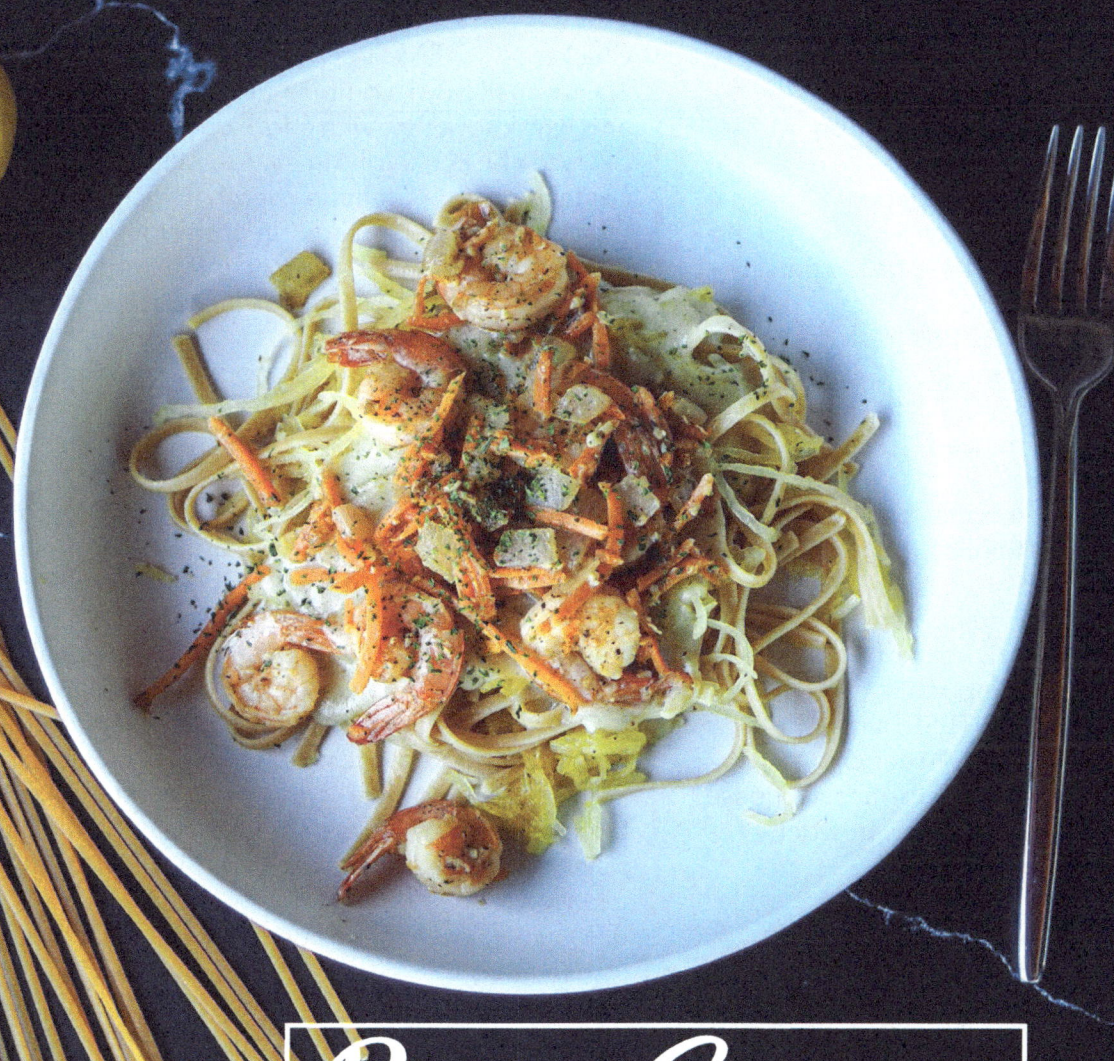

Part Seven:
DINNER

HERBED CHICKEN WITH MASHED CAULI

SERVINGS: 4   MAKES: 4 THIGHS, 1 1/2 CUP CAULI   TIME: 50 MINUTES

INGREDIENTS:

Marinade:
2 TBSP olive oil
Juice of 1 lemon
1/2 tsp salt
1/2 tsp pepper
3-4 cloves garlic, minced
1-2 TBSP Italian parsley, minced
1-2 TBSP fresh rosemary, minced
1-2 TBSP fresh thyme, minced

4 boneless, skinless chicken thighs

Cauliflower:
1/2 head of cauliflower, chopped
1/2 TBSP butter
1 TBSP sour cream
2 TBSP Parmesan cheese
1 tsp garlic powder
1/2 tsp salt
1/2 tsp pepper

● GENERAL DIET

DIRECTIONS:

Chicken:
1. In a small bowl, combine all marinade ingredients and whisk together with a fork until well combined.
2. Place chicken thighs in a large plastic bag or glass container. Pour marinade over the chicken; make sure the chicken is well-coated on both sides.
3. Close the plastic bag or cover the container with a lid or plastic wrap. Place in the refrigerator and marinate for 30 minutes or overnight.
4. Preheat a large pan over medium heat on the stove top. Place each chicken thigh on the hot pan and cook for 7-8 minutes per side or until the internal temperature of the chicken reaches 165 degrees F.

Cauliflower:
1. Fill a medium-sized pot with about 1 inch of water and place on medium-high heat on the stove top.
2. Add the cauliflower to the pot and cover. Bring the water to a boil and steam the cauliflower for about 5-6 minutes or until very soft.
7. Drain the cauliflower with a strainer and transfer to a blender or food processor. Add the butter, sour cream, Parmesan cheese, garlic powder, salt, and pepper to the blender/food processor. Blend until a smooth consistency. This recipe makes about 1 1/2 cups of mashed cauliflower.
8. To serve, include 1/3 cup mashed cauliflower and 1 chicken thigh.

Nutrition Facts (1 thigh + about 1/3 cup cauli):
313 calories, 30g protein, 4g carbohydrates, 20g fat

TIPS/SUGGESTIONS:
- Make the cauliflower while the chicken marinates in the refrigerator to save on time.

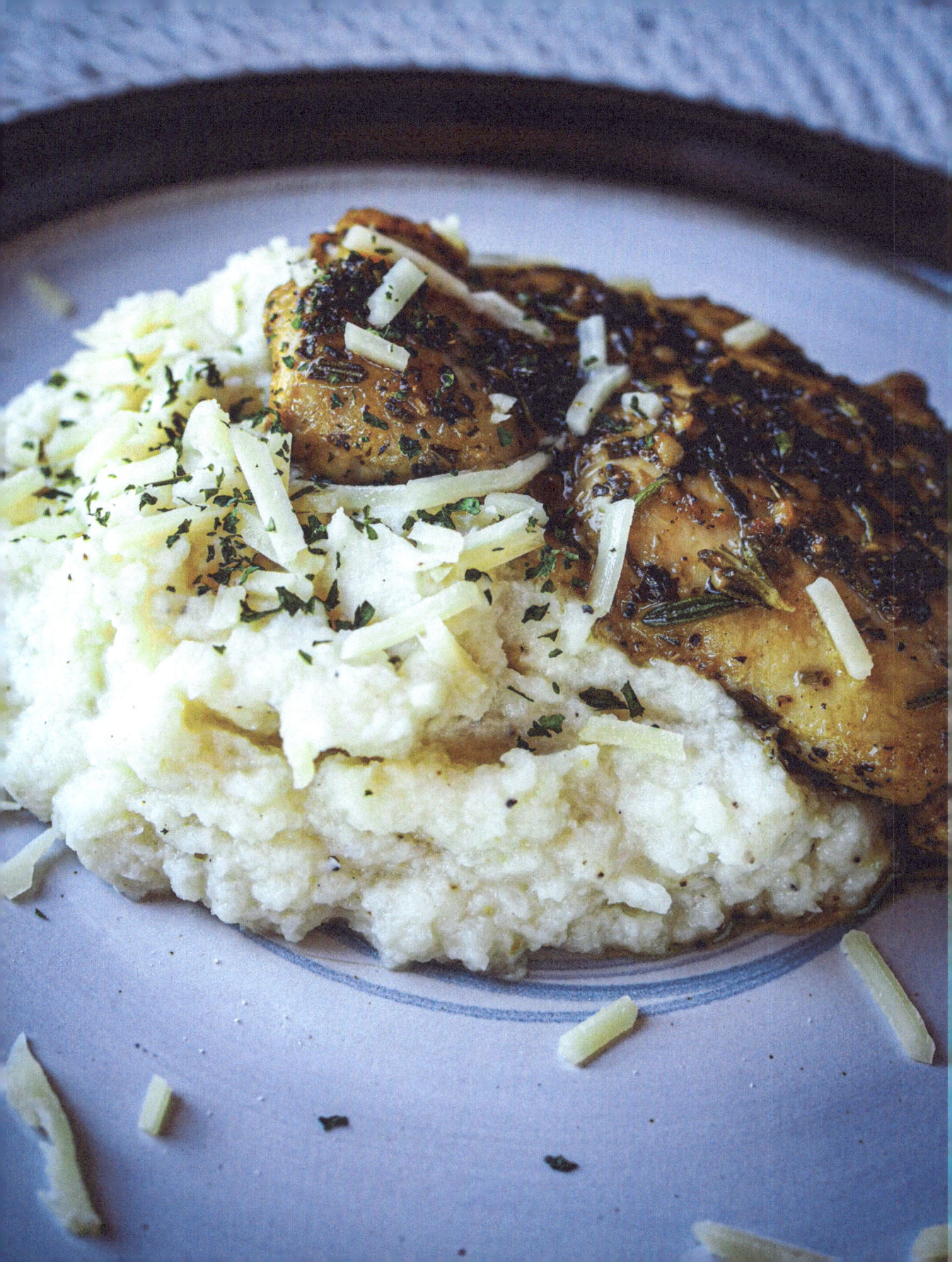

Part Seven: Dinner

TURKEY TACOS

SERVINGS: 5 **MAKES: 2 1/2 CUPS** **TIME: 40 MINUTES**

INGREDIENTS:

2 tsp olive oil
1/2 pound ground turkey
1/4 cup onion, diced
3 cloves garlic, minced
1/4 cup sweet potato, peeled and shredded (using a cheese grater)
1/2 cup shredded carrots
1/2 15.5-ounce can pinto beans, drained and rinsed
1/2 16-ounce can of salsa
1 tsp chili powder
1/4 tsp cumin
1/4 tsp salt

Optional ingredients:
Low carbohydrate tortillas
Romaine lettuce leaves
Shredded cheese
Shredded lettuce

DIRECTIONS:

1. Preheat olive oil in a large pan over medium heat on the stove top.
2. Add the ground turkey to the pan and using a wooden spoon break up the turkey into small pieces and cook until browned and cooked through.
3. Add the onion, garlic, sweet potato, carrots, pinto beans and salsa to the pan. While stirring occasionally bring the mixture to a boil and cook until the vegetables begin to soften and most of the liquid is evaporated, about 5-7 minutes.
4. Mix in the chili powder, cumin, and salt. Cook for an additional 5-7 minutes.
5. Remove the pan from the heat and allow to cool for 5 minutes before using in a taco, taco salad, or by itself.

● GENERAL DIET

Nutrition Facts (1/2 cup):
144 calories, 12g protein, 13g carbohydrates, 5g fat

TIPS/SUGGESTIONS:
- You can include these with a low carbohydrate tortilla, put this in a lettuce wrap or include this meat mixture over lettuce to make a taco salad.
- The nutrition info does not include any optional ingredients.

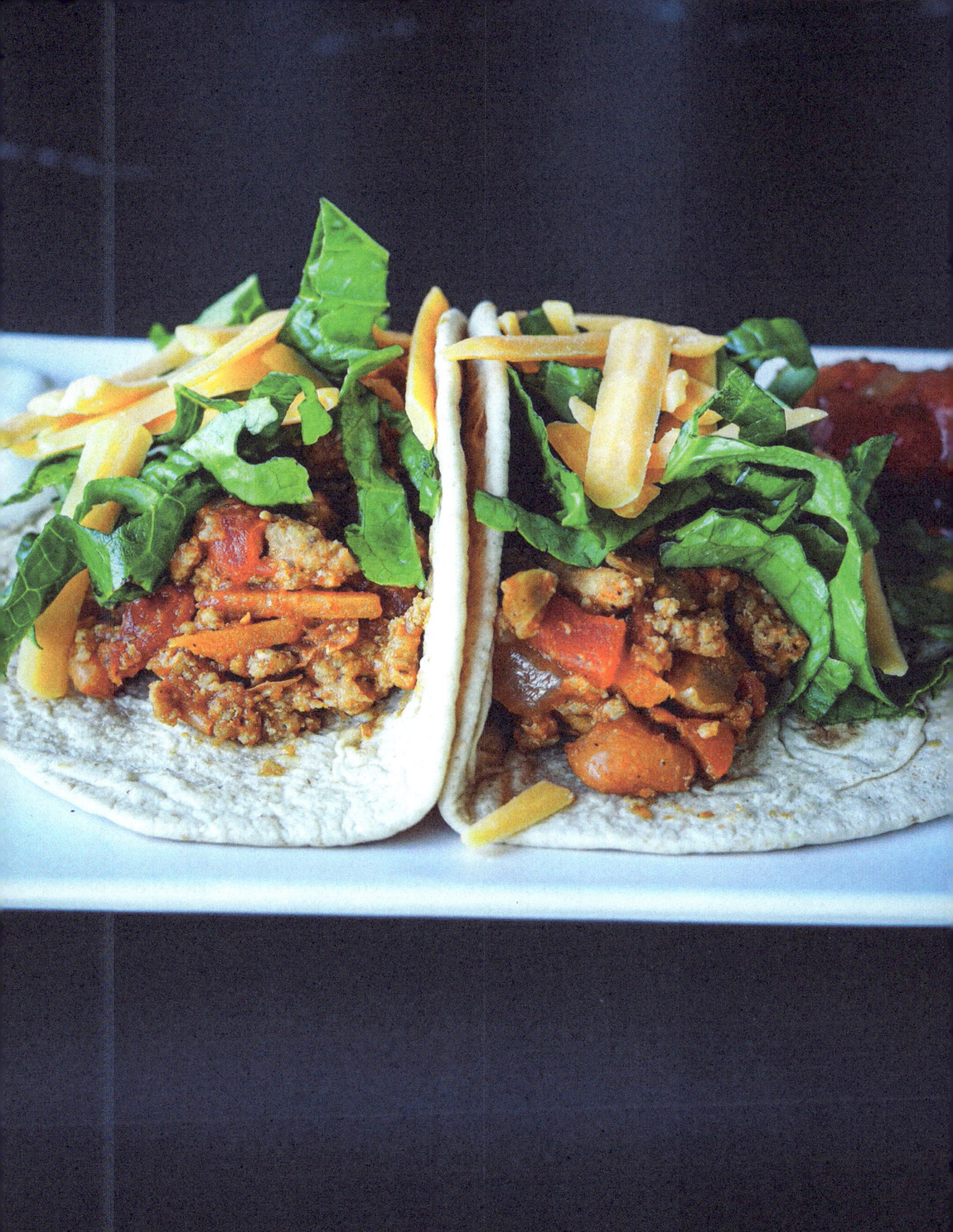

Part Seven: Dinner

STUFFED PORK CHOPS

SERVINGS: 2 **MAKES: 2 PORK CHOPS** **TIME: 45 MINUTES**

INGREDIENTS:

4 stems broccolini or asparagus spears, ends trimmed
2 tsp olive oil, divided
4-ounce boneless pork chop, fat trimmed
1/4 tsp salt, plus more to taste
1/4 tsp pepper, plus more to taste
1/8 tsp dried sage
1/4 tsp garlic powder
1 TBSP tomato pesto
2 cloves garlic, minced
2 TBSP shredded mozzarella cheese
1/4 cup spinach leaves, chopped and packed

● GENERAL DIET

TIPS/SUGGESTIONS:
- Set up and measure out ingredients first for an easier assembly of the pork.
- Wash hands well under hot water after handling raw meat.

DIRECTIONS:

1. Preheat oven to 375 degrees F. Preheat 1 tsp olive oil in a small pan over medium heat on the stove top.
2. Prepare a small baking sheet by lining it with tin foil.
3. Add broccolini or asparagus to the hot pan on the stove top, cooking for 2 minutes per side. Add salt and pepper to taste.
4. Remove broccolini or asparagus from heat and set aside on a plate.
5. Preheat 1 tsp olive oil in the same small pan over medium heat on the stove top.
6. While the oil is preheating prepare the pork chops.
7. Slice the pork chop in half to create two separate 2 ounce pork chops. Butterfly each pork chop half.
8. Combine salt, pepper, sage, and garlic powder in a small bowl. Sprinkle half of this mixture over each pork chop, and using your hands, rub an even layer onto all side of the pork.
9. Open up each pork chop, spread 1/2 TBSP tomato pesto, and 1 garlic clove on the inside. Sprinkle with 1 TBSP mozzarella cheese, 1/8 cup of spinach leaves, then lay the asparagus or broccolini over top of the spinach.
10. Roll up the pork chop and secure with 2-3 toothpicks.
11. Place each pork chop on the hot skillet and cook each side for 3-4 minutes. Each side should be brown and crisp. Remove toothpicks from the pork.
12. Transfer the pork to the baking sheet, cover with tin foil, and cook in the oven for 15 minutes. Remove from the oven and let sit for 10 minutes; make sure the pork reaches an internal temperature of 145 degrees F. Serve with additional vegetables, cauliflower rice, or salad.

Nutrition Facts (1/2 of recipe, 2 ounce pork chop):
232 calories, 18g protein, 2g carbohydrates, 17g fat

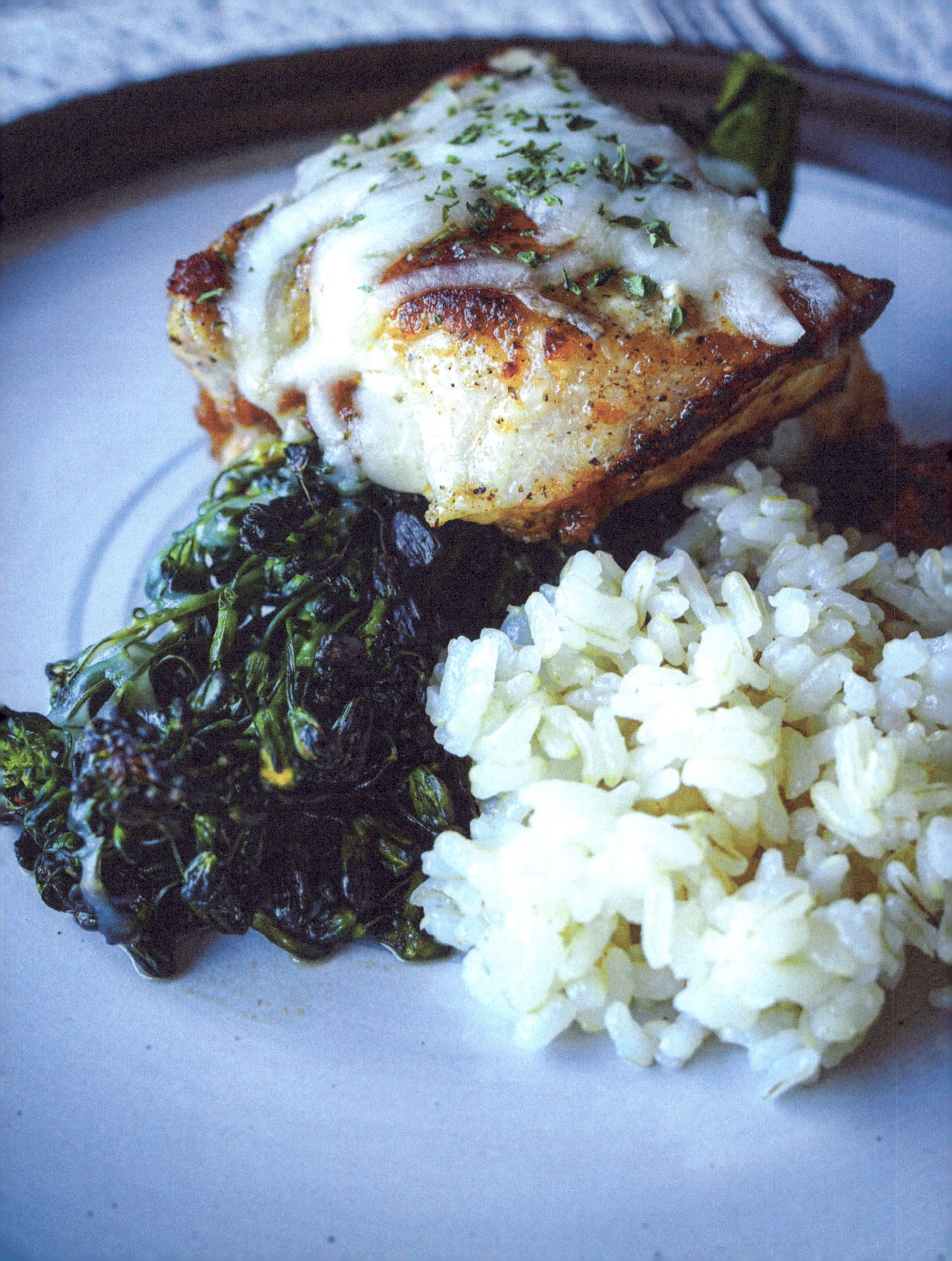

BLACK BEAN SWEET POTATO TACOS

SERVINGS: 2-4 **MAKES: 4 TACOS** **TIME: 35 MINUTES**

INGREDIENTS:

2-3 tsp olive oil, divided
1/2 cup red bell pepper, diced
1/4 cup shredded carrots
1/4 cup onion, diced
2-3 cloves garlic, minced
1/4 cup sweet potatoes, peeled and diced
1/4 cup canned black beans, drained and rinsed
1/4 tsp salt
1/4 tsp cumin
1/2 tsp chili powder
1/4 cup avocado, diced
1/4 cup tomatoes, diced
1/4 cup queso fresco, crumbled
4 corn tortillas

Optional ingredients:
Salsa
Cilantro
Hot sauce

DIRECTIONS:

1. Preheat 2 tsp olive oil in a large pan over medium heat on the stove top.
2. Add the bell pepper, carrots, onion, garlic, and sweet potatoes to the hot pan. Stir the vegetables until they are well-coated in the oil then cover the pan. Allow the vegetables to cook until soft, about 8-10 minutes while stirring occasionally. The sweet potatoes may take a little longer to soften; check them by piercing with a fork.
3. Add the black beans, salt, cumin, and chili powder to the pan. Add another 1 tsp of olive oil if the mixture is getting dry. Cook for an additional 2-3 minutes.
4. Remove the pan from the heat and assemble the tacos. Stuff each corn tortilla with 1/4 of the mixture in the pan, 1 TBSP avocado, 1 TBSP tomatoes, and 1 TBSP queso fresco.

● **GENERAL DIET**

Nutrition Facts (1 taco):
177 calories, 8g protein, 22g carbohydrates, 6g fat

TIPS/SUGGESTIONS:
- This recipe pairs well with the fiesta rice (on page 90), a side salad or roasted vegetables.

Part Seven: Dinner

VEGETARIAN BOLOGNESE

SERVINGS: 4 **MAKES: ABOUT 2 CUPS** **TIME: 40 MINUTES**

INGREDIENTS:

2 tsp olive oil
1/2 cup onion, diced
1/2 cup celery, diced
1/2 cup carrots, peeled and diced
4-5 cloves garlic, minced
1/4 cup walnuts, chopped- (general diet only)
1 TBSP tomato paste
1 cup canned lentils, drained and rinsed
1 tsp Italian seasoning
1 tsp salt
1/2 can diced tomatoes (with their juices)
1 cup vegetable broth or beef broth
1/4 cup 2% milk

DIRECTIONS:

1. Preheat olive oil in a large pan over medium-high heat on the stove top.
2. Add onion, celery, carrots and garlic to the pan. Stir until the vegetables are well-coated in the oil and cook for 7-8 minutes or until the vegetables begin to soften, continuing to stir occasionally.
3. Add the walnuts (general diet only), tomato paste, canned lentils and Italian seasoning to the pan. Stir the mixture until it is well combined and cook for 2-3 minutes.
4. Add the canned tomatoes and broth, bring the mixture to a boil and cover. Reduce heat to low and allow the mixture to simmer for 15-20 minutes or until the vegetables are soft while continuing to stir occasionally. If you are using this recipe on a soft foods diet cook the vegetables until very soft and well-done.
5. Uncover the pot and slowly stir in the milk. Bring the mixture to a low boil again and stir continuously until half of the liquid is evaporated or the Bolognese reaches the consistency you desire.

- SOFT FOODS DIET
- GENERAL DIET

Nutrition Facts (1/2 cup):
169 calories, 7g protein, 20g carbohydrates, 7g fat

TIPS/SUGGESTIONS:
- You can eat this Bolognese by itself or serve over cottage cheese for additional protein. You can also serve with zucchini spirals.
- Do not include the walnuts if you are enjoying this recipe on a soft foods diet.

Part Seven: Dinner

TURKEY & VEGETABLE MEATBALLS

SERVINGS: 5 **MAKES: 10 MEATBALLS** **TIME: 55 MINUTES**

INGREDIENTS:

1/2 pound ground turkey
1/2 pound ground turkey sausage
1 tsp salt
1 tsp pepper
4 cloves garlic, minced
1/4 tsp sage
1/4 tsp parsley
1/4 cup Parmesan cheese
2 TBSP bread crumbs
1/2 large carrot, shredded
1/2 large zucchini, shredded

DIRECTIONS:

1. Preheat oven to 425 degrees F and line a large baking sheet with tin foil.
2. Mix turkey and turkey sausage in a large bowl until well combined.
3. Add salt, pepper, garlic, sage, parsley, Parmesan cheese and bread crumbs. Shred carrot and zucchini with cheese shredder and add to the bowl.
4. Mix all ingredients together with a wooden spoon or your hands. Using a 1/4 measuring cup, scoop the mixture, and roll into meatballs using your hands. This makes approximately ten 2-ounce meatballs. You can also use a food scale to measure about 2 ounces for each meatball.
5. Place each meatball on the baking sheet, making sure they are spread out by about 1-2 inches. Wash your hands well with hot water after handling raw poultry.
6. Place the meatballs in the oven and bake for 40 minutes or until the internal temperature reaches 165 degrees F.

Nutrition Facts (1 meatball):
86 calories, 10g protein, 1g carbohydrate, 5g fat

● GENERAL DIET

TIPS/SUGGESTIONS:
- Enjoy these meatballs with some marinara, leafy greens and roasted vegetables, include with some spaghetti squash for a low carbohydrate spaghetti recipe, or they make a great high-protein snack between meals.

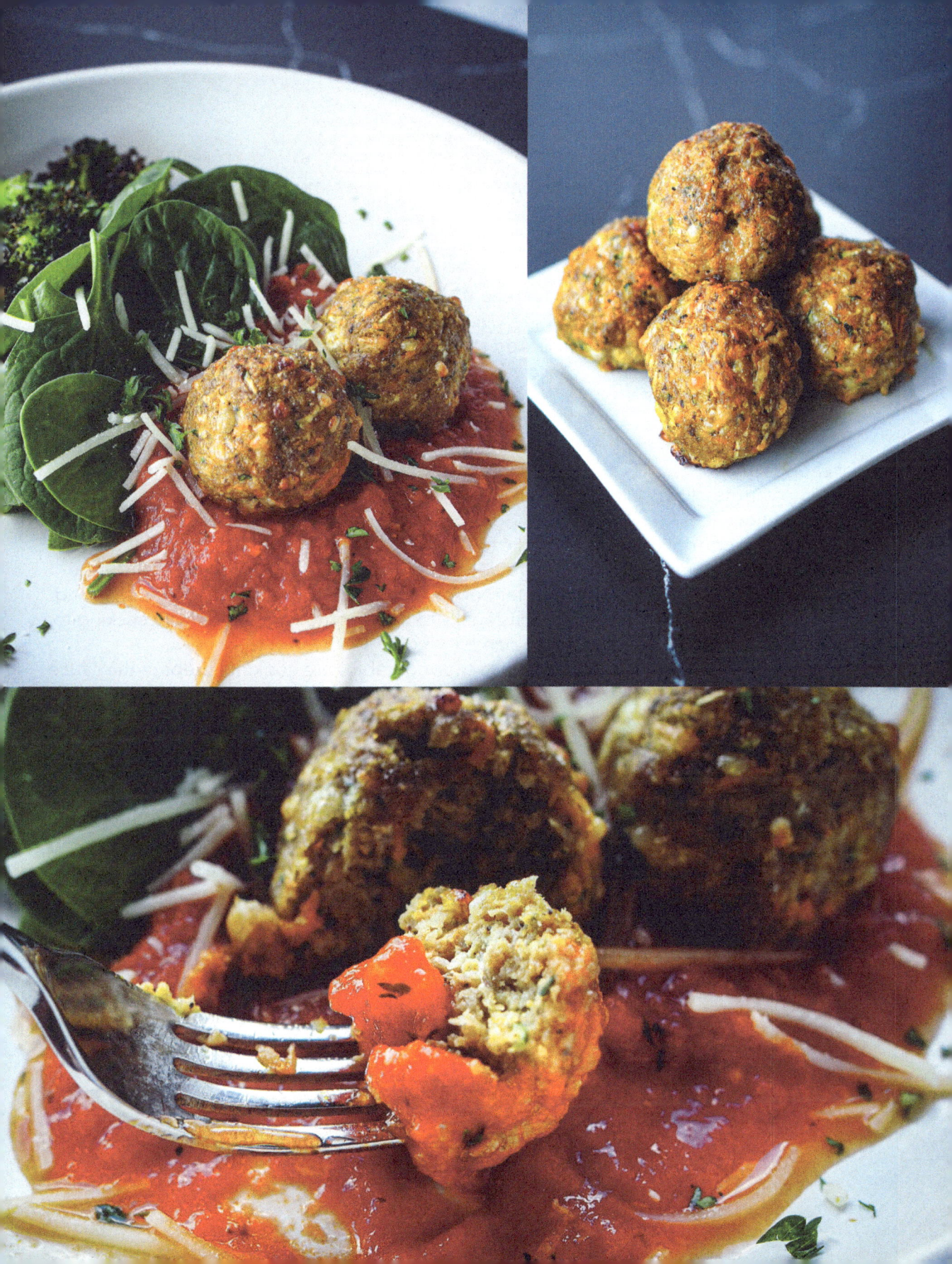

Part Seven: Dinner

BEEF & VEGETABLE TERIYAKI

SERVINGS: 4 **MAKES: ABOUT 4 CUPS** **TIME: 40 MINUTES**

INGREDIENTS:

12 ounces lean steak, sliced in strips
1/2 tsp garlic powder
1/2 tsp ground ginger
Salt/pepper, to taste
1 TBSP sesame oil
2 cups broccoli florets, chopped
1 cup carrots, sliced
1 cup snow peas
1/2 bell pepper, sliced
3 cloves garlic, minced
1/2 cup soy sauce
1 1/2 TBSP brown sugar, packed
1 TBSP corn starch

Optional ingredients:
1/2 tsp sesame seeds
1/2 cup brown rice or cauliflower rice, cooked

DIRECTIONS:

1. Preheat a large nonstick pan over medium heat on the stove top.
2. Add strips of steak to the pan and season with garlic powder, ginger, salt, and pepper. Continue cooking for about 5-6 minutes per side or until steak is cooked through. Transfer the steak to a small plate and set aside.
4. Preheat sesame oil in the same pan over medium heat.
5. Add broccoli, carrots, snow peas, bell pepper, and garlic to the hot pan. Give it a good stir to coat the vegetables in the sesame oil then cover. Let the vegetables cook while covered for about 5 minutes, stirring occasionally to prevent the vegetables from sticking to the pan.
6. While the vegetables are cooking, prepare the sauce. Using a liquid measuring cup combine soy sauce, brown sugar, and corn starch. Whisk together until smooth.
7. Uncover the pan and continue cooking until any liquid is evaporated. Return steak to the pan and cook with the vegetables for 2 minutes, stirring frequently.
8. Slowly add the sauce to the pan and cook until the sauce thickens, about 1-2 minutes while continuing to stir frequently. The sauce will thicken quickly.
9. Remove the pan from the heat and allow to cook for about 5 minutes before dishing up.

● GENERAL DIET

Nutrition Facts (1/4 of recipe, about 1 cup):
328 calories, 28g protein, 18.5g carbohydrates, 17g fat

TIPS/SUGGESTIONS:
- Don't be too concerned about the brown sugar in this recipe. You can consider sugar like a condiment and sometimes condiments are needed to enjoy healthy foods and your healthy diet.

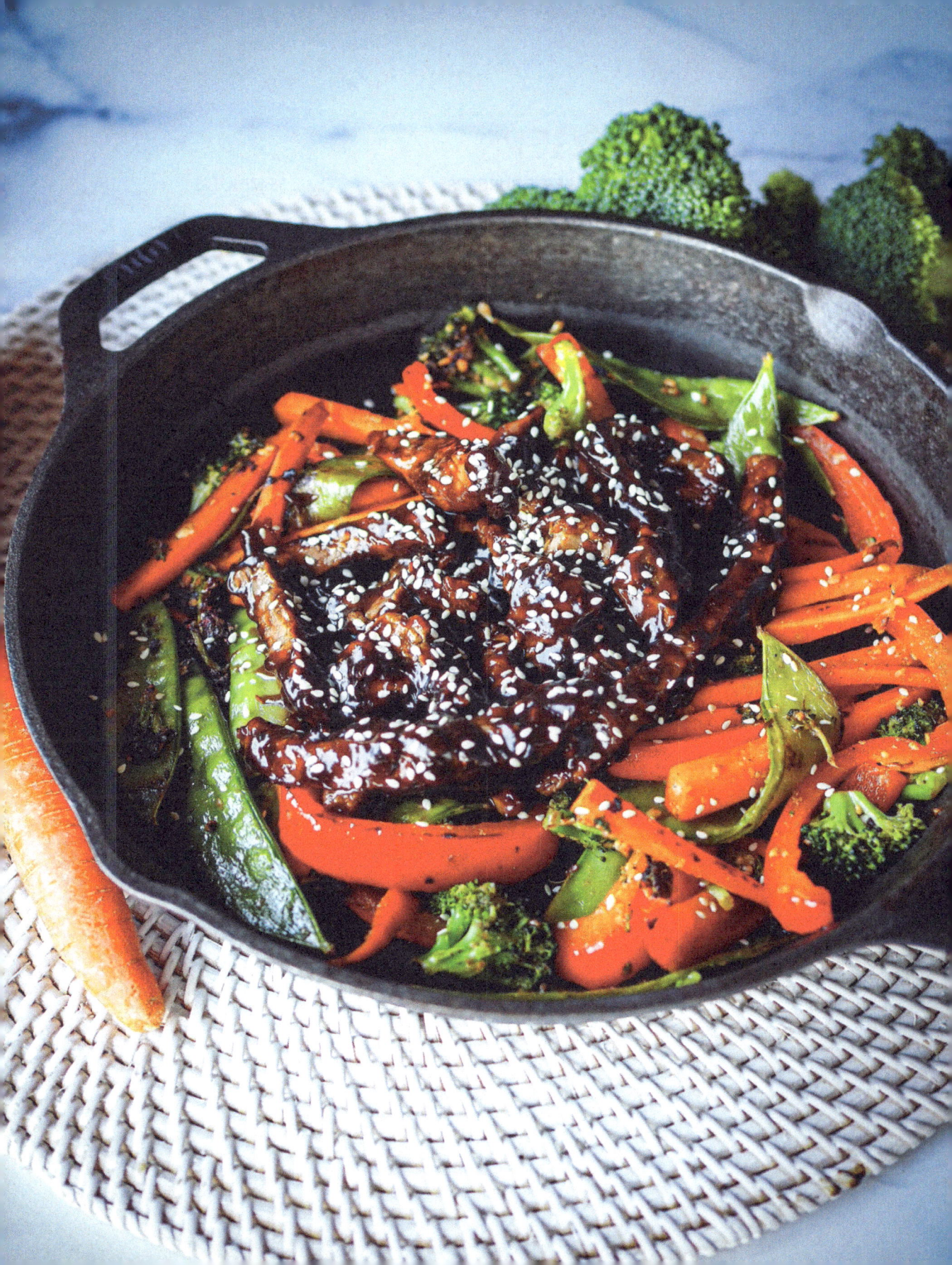

Part Seven: Dinner

CHICKEN BURGERS

SERVINGS: 5 **MAKES: 5 BURGERS** **TIME: 35 MINUTES**

INGREDIENTS:

1 tsp olive oil
1/2 pound ground chicken
1/4 cup bread crumbs
1/4 cup feta cheese, crumbled
1 TBSP basil pesto
1 tsp garlic powder
1/4 tsp salt
1/4 tsp pepper
1/4 tsp Italian seasoning
1/2 cup canned cannellini beans, drained, rinsed and mashed with a fork
1/2 small zucchini, shredded

DIRECTIONS:

1. Preheat olive oil in a large pan over medium heat on the stove top.
2. In a medium-sized mixing bowl, combine ground chicken, bread crumbs, feta cheese, basil pesto, garlic powder, salt, pepper, Italian seasoning, mashed cannellini beans and zucchini.
3. Using a wooden spoon or your hands, mix the ingredients together until well combined. Make sure to wash your hands well with hot water after touching raw poultry.
4. Taking about 3 ounces of the chicken mixture, roll into a ball, then flatten with your hands to create a burger. This recipe makes about five 3-ounce burgers.
5. Place each burger on the hot pan and cook for about 8-10 minutes on each side or until the internal temperature reaches 165 degrees F.

● **GENERAL DIET**

Nutrition Facts (1 burger, about 3 ounces):
139 calories, 13g protein, 9g carbohydrates, 6g fat

TIPS/SUGGESTIONS:
- Serve these chicken burgers with your favorite salad or pair with roasted vegetables for a balanced meal.
- Make ahead of time and store them in the refrigerator for up to three to four days to have a quick meal ready to go.

BURRITO BOWLS

SERVINGS: 2 **MAKES: 1 1/2-2 CUPS** **TIME: 20 MINUTES**

INGREDIENTS:

4 ounces chicken breast, cooked and shredded
1 tsp chili powder
1 tsp cumin
Salt/pepper to taste
1/4 cup quinoa, cooked
1/4 cup canned black beans, drained and rinsed
1/4 cup mashed avocado
2 TBSP salsa
2 TBSP sour cream

Optional ingredients (general diet only):
2 TBSP cilantro leaves, chopped
2 TBSP bell pepper, diced
2 TBSP red onion, diced

DIRECTIONS:

1. In a small bowl, mix together the chicken, chili powder, cumin and salt/pepper to taste.
2. In two separate small bowls, add 2 ounces of the seasoned chicken, 2 TBSP quinoa, 2 TBSP black beans, 2 TBSP mashed avocado, 1 TBSP salsa, and 1 TBSP sour cream.
4. Mix together with a fork or spoon and add additional salt, pepper, or optional ingredients if you would like. Please note the optional ingredients are for those who are on a general diet.

- SOFT FOODS DIET
- GENERAL DIET

Nutrition Facts (1/2 of recipe, measured as recommended in step 2):
212 calories, 17g protein, 16g carbohydrates, 15.5g fat

TIPS/SUGGESTIONS:
- The nutrition facts do not include the optional ingredients.
- Once you have advanced to a general diet get creative and add your favorite vegetables. Just make sure to adjust the nutrition facts as needed.

Part Seven: Dinner
COCONUT CHICKEN CURRY

SERVINGS: 5   **MAKES: 5 CUPS**   **TIME: 45 MINUTES**

INGREDIENTS:

1 TBSP coconut oil, divided
2 large chicken breasts (about 6-8 ounces each), diced
2 cloves garlic, minced
1/2 onion, chopped
1/2 head cauliflower florets, chopped
1/2 red bell pepper, sliced
1 15 ounce can diced tomatoes
1 tsp salt
1/2 tsp pepper
1 tsp garlic powder
1 TBSP curry powder
1 tsp ground ginger
1/2 tsp coriander
1/2 can lite coconut milk

Optional ingredients:
1.5 cup brown rice
Cilantro

DIRECTIONS:

1. Preheat 1/2 TBSP of coconut oil in a large pan over medium heat on the stove top.
2. Add the chicken to the pan and cook until the chicken is cooked through, about 8 minutes while stirring occasionally. Transfer the chicken to a small plate and set aside.
3. Preheat 1/2 TBSP of coconut oil in the same pan over medium heat on the stove top. Add the garlic, onion, cauliflower, and bell pepper. While stirring occasionally allow the vegetable mixture to cook until the vegetables begin to soften, about 6-8 minutes.
4. Add the chicken, canned tomatoes, salt, pepper, garlic powder, curry powder, ground ginger, and coriander to the pan. Stir well. Cover the pan and allow the mixture to cook for an additional 8-10 minutes or until the vegetables are soft, stirring occasionally.
5. Uncover and add the coconut milk. Bring the mixture to a boil, then lower the temperature to allow the mixture to simmer for another 10-15 minutes or until the desired amount of liquid has evaporated (some people like more soup-ier curries than others).
6. Remove the pan from the heat and allow to cool for 5 minutes.
7. Serve over brown rice or cauliflower rice and garnish with fresh cilantro if you would like.

● GENERAL DIET

Nutrition Facts (1/5 of recipe, 1 cup):
170 calories, 17g protein, 8g carbohydrates, 7g fat

TIPS/SUGGESTIONS:
- To make this recipe vegetarian replace the chicken with 1 can of garbanzo beans, drained and rinsed.

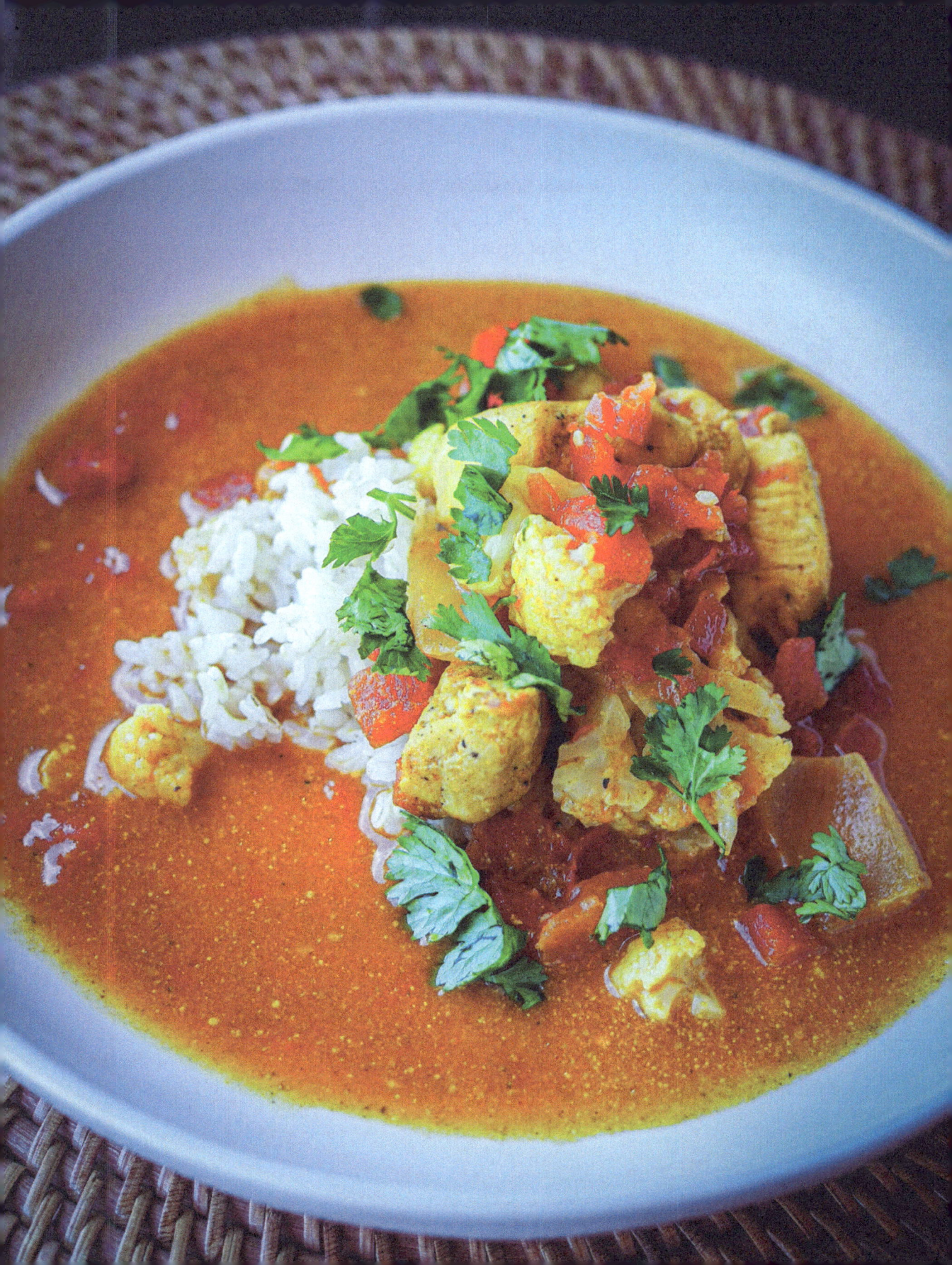

SHEPHERD'S PIE

SERVINGS: 6 **MAKES: 1 LARGE PIE** **TIME: 50 MINUTES**

INGREDIENTS:

1/2 head cauliflower florets, chopped
1/2 pound lean ground beef
1/2 cup onion, diced
1/2 cup carrots, peeled and diced
1/2 cup parsnips, peeled and diced
3/4 tsp salt
1/2 tsp pepper
1 TBSP Worcestershire sauce
1/2 cup zucchini, diced
1 cup canned lentils, drained and rinsed
3/4 cup beef broth, divided
1/2 tsp dried rosemary
1/2 tsp dried thyme
1/2 tsp dried sage
1 TBSP cornstarch
1/4 cup 1% milk
1 TBSP butter

● GENERAL DIET

DIRECTIONS:

1. Preheat oven to 425 degrees F.
2. Fill a medium-sized pot with about 1 inch of water and place on medium-high heat on the stove top. Add the cauliflower to the pot and cover. Steam the cauliflower until soft enough to be pierced by a fork and then remove from heat and use a strainer to remove the liquid. Set the cauliflower aside.
3. Preheat a large pan over medium heat on the stove top. Add the ground beef and cook until browned, breaking up the meat with a spatula into small pieces.
4. Add the onion, carrots, and parsnips to the pan and cook until the vegetables begin to soften, about 6-8 minutes. Add the salt, pepper, Worcestershire sauce, zucchini, lentils, 1/4 cup broth, rosemary, thyme, and sage. Cover the pan, bring to a boil and allow the mixture to cook for about 5-6 minutes or until the liquid is evaporated.
5. Uncover the pot and add 1/2 cup beef broth and 1 TBSP cornstarch. Bring mixture to a boil and cover again, allowing it to cook for another 4-5 minutes.
6. Transfer mixture to a pie dish or an 8x8 baking dish and spread out into an even layer.
7. Prepare the cauliflower: Using a blender or food processor, blend the cauliflower, milk, and butter until a smooth consistency.
8. Spread the cauliflower over top of the beef and lentil mixture into an even layer. Place the baking dish in the oven and bake for 20 minutes. Remove the pan from the oven and allow to cool for about 5 minutes before serving.

Nutrition Facts (1/6 of pie):
154 calories, 12g protein, 15g carbohydrates, 6g fat

BEAN, SAUSAGE & VEGGIE SKILLET

SERVINGS: 4 **MAKES: 4 CUPS** **TIME: 30 MINUTES**

INGREDIENTS:

1 TBSP olive oil
1/2 small white onion, sliced
2 celery stalks, chopped
1 cup cabbage, shredded
1/2 green bell pepper, sliced
4-5 cloves garlic, minced
1/2 14-ounce can of diced tomatoes, including juices
1/2 15.5-ounce can of kidney beans, drained and rinsed
1/2 tsp salt
1/4 tsp pepper
1/2 tsp dried sage
1/4 tsp paprika
2 lean Cajun sausage links (fully cooked), diced

Optional ingredient:
Brown rice

DIRECTIONS:

1. Preheat olive oil in a large pan over medium heat on the stove top.
2. Add the onion, celery, cabbage, bell pepper and garlic to the pan. Cook the vegetables for about 4-5 minutes or until they begin to soften, stirring occasionally.
3. Add the tomatoes, kidney beans, salt, pepper, sage and paprika to the pan. Cover and cook for 4-5 minutes.
4. Uncover the pot and add the sausage links. Continue to stir occasionally and let the mixture cook for another 7-8 minutes or until the sausages are heated through.
5. Remove the pan from the heat and allow to cool for about 5 minutes before serving.
5. You can include a couple of tablespoons of brown rice if you would like to, and you are done!

● GENERAL DIET

Nutrition Facts (1/4 of recipe, 1 cup):
191 calories, 12g protein, 16g carbohydrates, 9g fat

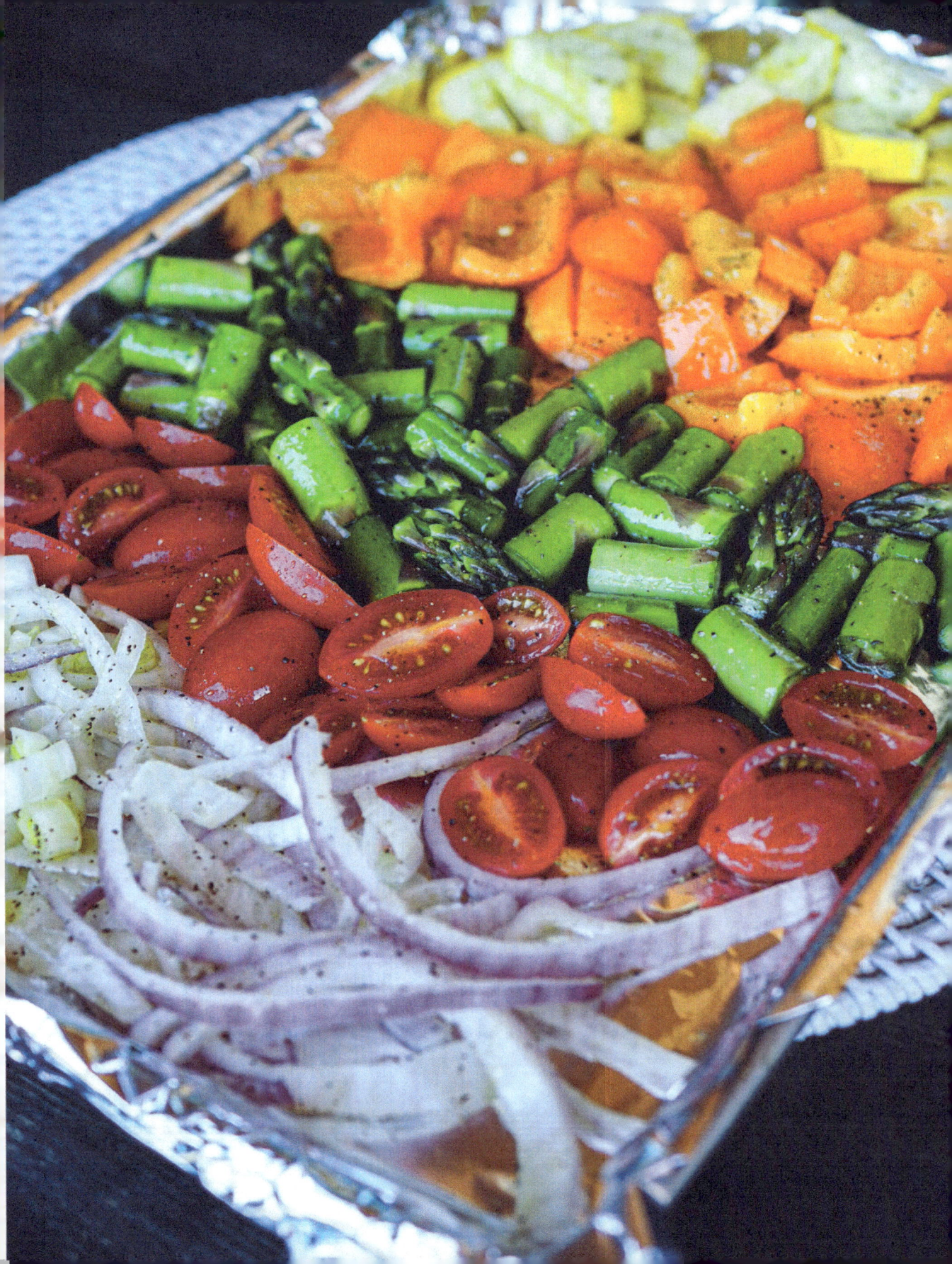

ROASTED VEGETABLE PASTA SALAD

SERVINGS: 4   **MAKES: ABOUT 4 CUPS**   **TIME: 30 MINUTES**

INGREDIENTS:

1 cup penne pasta, cooked and cooled
1/2 cup red onion, sliced
1 bell pepper, chopped
1/2 cup asparagus, ends removed and chopped
1/2 cup cherry tomatoes, sliced in half
1/2 cup summer squash, chopped
1 TBSP olive oil
1 tsp salt
1 tsp pepper
1 TBSP pesto
1 TBSP Parmesan cheese
1 clove garlic

Optional topping:
2oz protein (chicken, fish, etc.)

DIRECTIONS:

1. Preheat oven to 425 degrees and line a large baking sheet with tin foil.
2. Combine red onion, bell pepper, asparagus, cherry tomatoes, and summer squash in a large bowl. Drizzle vegetables with olive oil, salt, and pepper. Mix until well combined.
3. Lay out vegetables on the baking sheet and spread out to make an even layer.
4. Place baking sheet in the oven and roast vegetables for about 15 minutes (stir vegetables half way through cooking).
5. Remove from oven and let vegetables cool to room temperature.
6. While vegetables are cooling, combine pasta, pesto, Parmesan cheese and garlic in a large bowl. Stir well.
7. Once vegetables are cooled add to the pasta mixture and mix together with a large wooden spoon.
8. Add your favorite protein to this pasta salad to create a light balanced meal. Perfect for the spring or summertime!

● GENERAL DIET

Nutrition Facts (1 cup):
135 calories, 5g protein, 17g carbohydrates, 6g fat

TIPS/SUGGESTIONS:
- The nutrition facts above do not include an added protein source.
- This recipe pairs great with fish like salmon, cod, or halibut.
- Sometimes pasta is not well tolerated for a few months after surgery; keep this in mind and monitor your tolerance.

TORTILLA-LESS CHICKEN ENCHILADAS

SERVINGS: 4 **MAKES: 4 ENCHILADAS** **TIME: 45 MINUTES**

INGREDIENTS:

1 TBSP olive oil
1/4 cup onion, diced
1/4 cup shredded zucchini
1/4 cup shredded carrots
1/2 bell pepper, diced
1/2 4 ounce can diced green chiles
3 cloves garlic, minced
1 cup chicken, cooked and shredded
1/2 cup canned black beans, drained and rinsed
19 ounce can red enchilada sauce, divided
1/2 tsp salt
1/4 tsp pepper
1/2 cup shredded Monterey Jack cheese, divided
4 savoy cabbage leaves

● GENERAL DIET

DIRECTIONS:

1. Preheat oven to 375 degrees F. Preheat olive oil in a large pan over medium heat on the stove top.
2. Add the onion, zucchini, carrots, bell pepper, green chiles and garlic to the pan. While stirring occasionally allow the mixture to cook for about 6-8 minutes or until the vegetables begin to soften.
3. Add the shredded chicken, black beans, 1/2 cup enchilada sauce, salt, and pepper to the pan. Continue to stir occasionally and allow the mixture to cook until most of the liquid has evaporated.
4. Remove the pan from the heat on the stove top and set aside.
5. Prepare a loaf pan by pouring a thin layer of enchilada sauce on the bottom of the pan.
6. Peel back a large savoy cabbage leaf and transfer about 1/2 cup of the chicken and vegetable mixture onto the leaf. Top with 1 TBSP cheese and then roll up the cabbage leaf and carefully place it into the loaf pan. You may need to tuck in the sides while rolling like you would a burrito.
7. Repeat this three to five more times with 3-5 more cabbage leaves until you have used up all of your chicken and vegetable mixture and your loaf pan is full.
8. Pour about 1/2-3/4 cup enchilada sauce over top of the enchiladas and sprinkle with the rest of the cheese.
9. Bake in the oven for 25 minutes or until the enchiladas are bubbly and the cabbage leaves are soft.

Nutrition Facts (1 enchilada):
240 calories, 16.5g protein, 20g carbohydrates, 9g fat

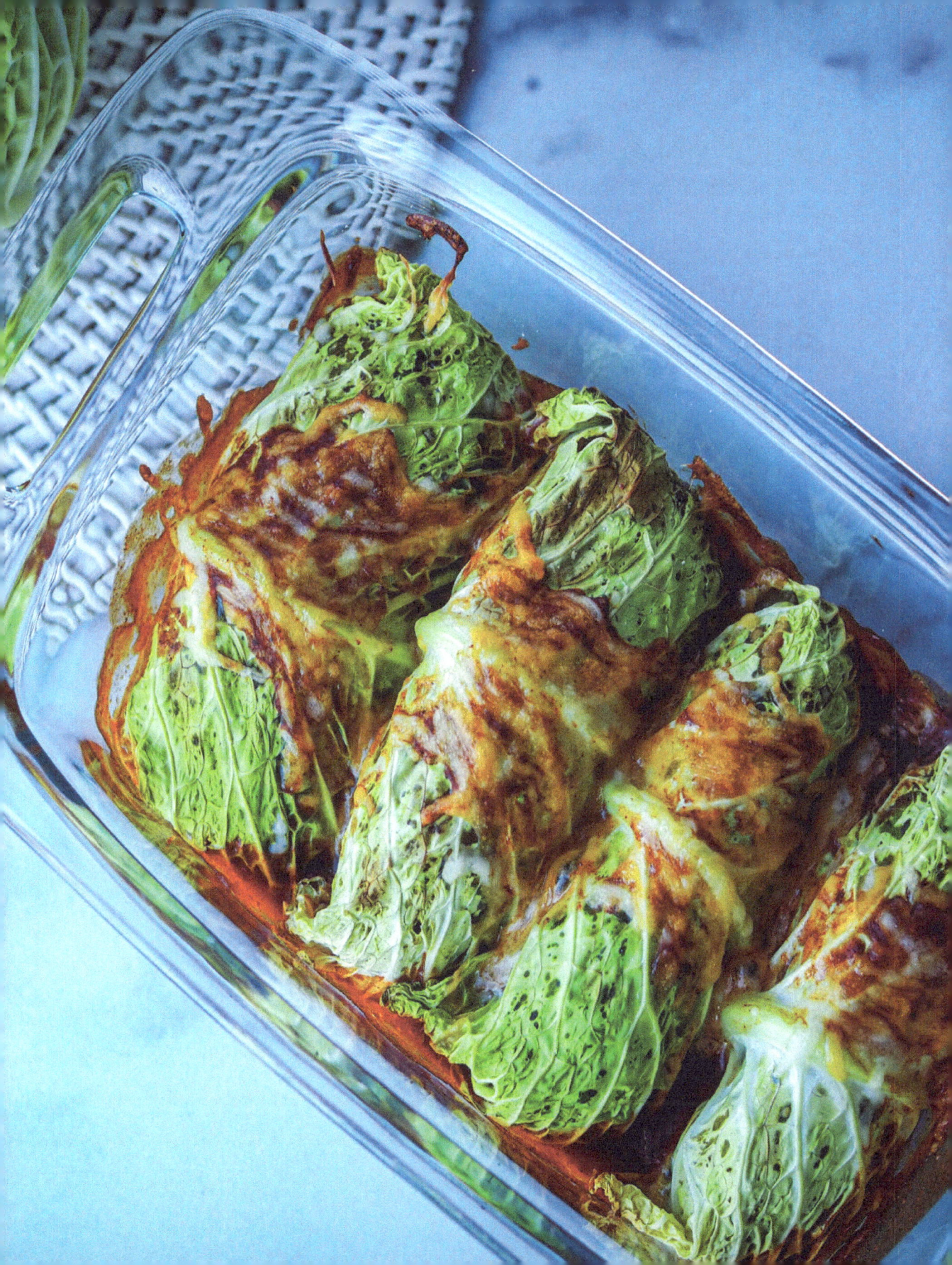

CHICKEN & BROCCOLI BAKE

SERVINGS: 4   **MAKES: ABOUT 4 CUPS**   **TIME: 45 MINUTES**

INGREDIENTS:

1 tsp olive oil
1 5.3-ounce container nonfat plain Greek yogurt
1 TBSP Dijon mustard
1/2 tsp salt
1/2 tsp pepper
1 tsp garlic powder
1/4 tsp cayenne pepper
1/4 tsp paprika
1 pound boneless skinless chicken breast, diced
1/4 cup onion, chopped
2 TBSP bread crumbs
1/2 cup shredded cheddar cheese
2 cups broccoli florets, chopped and steamed until soft

DIRECTIONS:

1. Preheat oven to 400 degrees F.
2. Preheat olive oil in a medium pan over medium heat on the stove top.
3. While the pan is preheating prepare the chicken. Combine yogurt, mustard, salt, pepper, garlic powder, cayenne pepper and paprika in a medium-sized bowl.
4. Add the chicken and stir until the chicken is well coated with the yogurt mixture.
5. Add the chicken to the pan and cook until liquid is mostly evaporated, approximately 15 minutes.
6. Add onion to the pan and cook for an additional 5 minutes.
7. Remove pan from heat and let it cool for 5 minutes.
8. Add breadcrumbs and broccoli to the pan and give it a couple of stirs.
9. Transfer mixture to an 8x8 baking dish. Top with cheddar cheese.
10. Bake in the oven at 400 degrees F for 15 minutes; remove from the oven and serve.

● GENERAL DIET

Nutrition Facts (1/4 of recipe, 1 cup):
232 calories, 28g protein, 9g carbohydrates, 9g fat

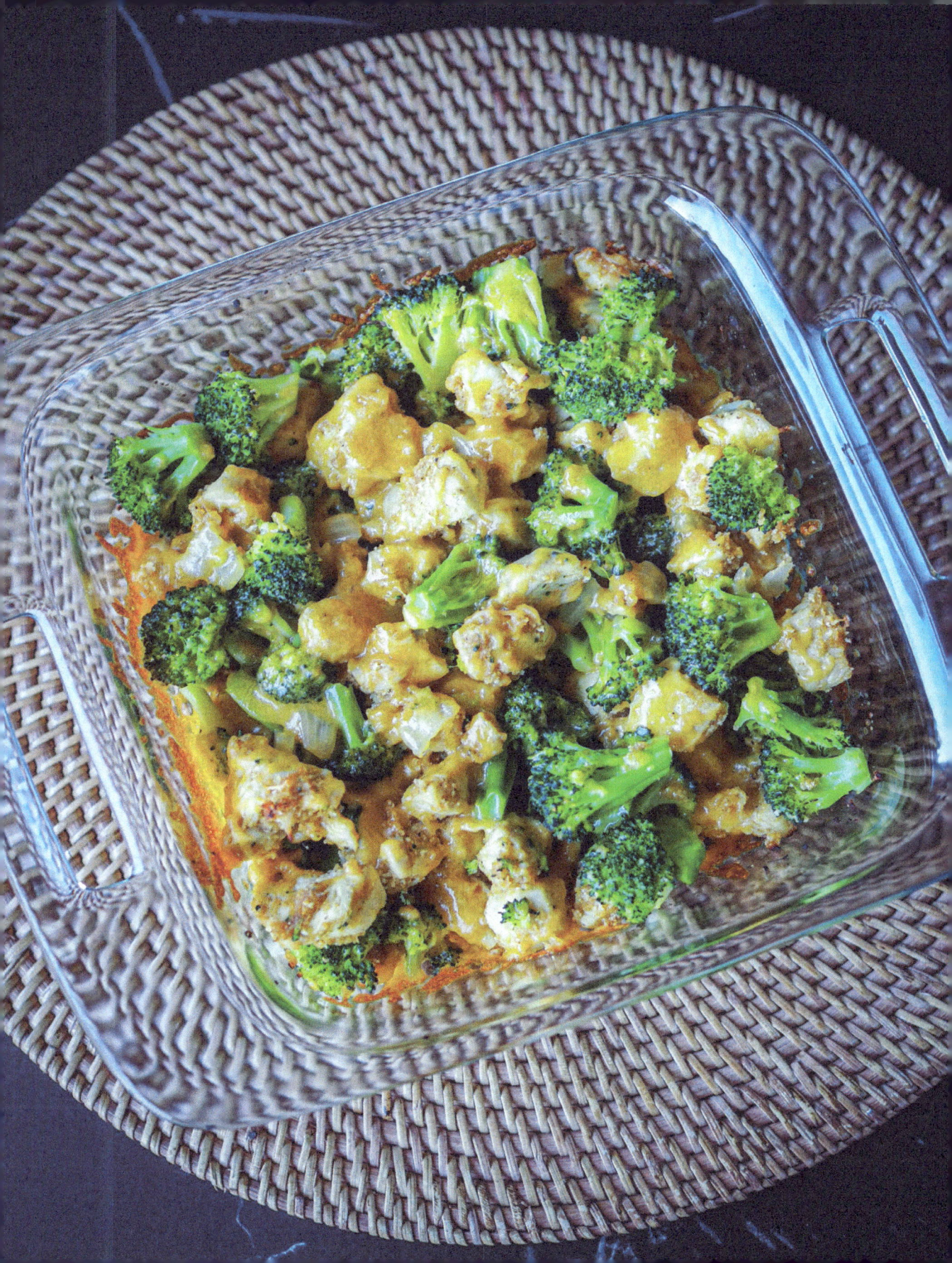

ONE PAN SALMON & BROCCOLI

SERVINGS: 2 **MAKES: 2 SERVINGS** **TIME: 35 MINUTES**

INGREDIENTS:

1 cup broccoli florets, chopped
1/2 cup red potatoes, diced
1 tsp olive oil
1/4 tsp salt
1/4 tsp pepper
1/2 tsp dried rosemary
1/2 tsp dried oregano
6 ounces salmon (two 3-ounce fillets, boneless and skin removed)
1 TBSP basil pesto

DIRECTIONS:

1. Preheat the oven to 400 degrees F and line a large baking sheet with tin foil.
2. Combine the broccoli, red potatoes, olive oil, salt, pepper, rosemary, and oregano in a medium mixing bowl. Mix together with a wooden spoon or clean hands until the vegetables are well coated with the herbs and oil.
3. Spread out the broccoli and red potatoes in an even layer on the baking sheet. Bake at 400 degrees F for 15 minutes.
4. Remove the pan from the oven and flip the potatoes and broccoli (I usually just give it a good toss and call it good). Make sure the vegetables are still spread out in an even layer on one side of the baking sheet.
5. Place the two salmon fillets on the same pan on the opposite side of the vegetables; top each fillet with 1/2 TBSP of basil pesto.
6. In order to prevent the fish from getting too dry, you can loosely cover the salmon fillets with tin foil.
7. Place the baking sheet back into the oven for 15 minutes; cook until the fish flakes easily and the vegetables are soft.

● GENERAL DIET

Nutrition Facts (3 ounces salmon + 1/3 cup vegetables):
280 calories, 20g protein, 10g carbohydrates, 17g fat

ONE PAN CHICKEN SAUSAGE & VEG

SERVINGS: 2 **MAKES: ABOUT 2 CUPS** **TIME: 40 MINUTES**

INGREDIENTS:

2 chicken sausage links, fully cooked and chopped
1/2 red bell pepper, chopped
1/2 cup shredded cabbage
1/4 cup onion, diced
1/2 cup carrots, peeled and diced
2 tsp olive oil
1/4 tsp salt
1/4 tsp pepper
1/2 tsp garlic powder

Optional ingredient:
1/4 cup cooked quinoa
2 TBSP mashed avocado

DIRECTIONS:

1. Preheat oven to 400 degrees F and line a large baking sheet with tin foil.
2. In a medium-sized bowl combine the sausage, bell pepper, cabbage, onion, carrots, olive oil, salt, pepper and garlic powder. Using a wooden spoon or clean hands, mix together until well combined.
3. Spread mixture into an even layer on the baking sheet and bake in the preheated oven for 25 minutes or until vegetables are soft.
4. Remove the pan from the oven and allow to cool for about 5 minutes before eating.

● GENERAL DIET

Nutrition Facts (1 cup chicken/veg mixture + 2 TBSP quinoa + 1 TBSP avocado):
284 calories, 16g protein, 16g carbohydrates, 18g fat

Part Seven: Dinner

STUFFED BELL PEPPERS

SERVINGS: 2   **MAKES: 2 PEPPERS**   **TIME: 50 MINUTES**

INGREDIENTS:

2 tsp olive oil, divided
1/4 cup onions, diced
3 cloves garlic, minced
4 ounces lean ground beef
1 large handful of fresh spinach leaves
1/4 cup zucchini, diced
1/2 cup canned cannellini beans, drained and rinsed
1/4 tsp salt
1/4 tsp pepper
1/4 tsp Italian seasoning
1/2 cup marinara sauce, divided
1 bell pepper, cut in half, seeds removed
2 TBSP Parmesan cheese, divided

● GENERAL DIET

DIRECTIONS:

1. Preheat oven to 425 degrees F. Preheat 1 tsp olive oil in a large pan over medium heat on the stove top.
2. Add onions and garlic to the pan and cook until fragrant, about 1-2 minutes. Add the ground beef to the pan, and using a wooden spoon, break up the ground beef until it's in small pieces and cook until browned.
3. Add the spinach, zucchini, white beans, salt, pepper, Italian seasoning, and 1/4 cup marinara to the pan. Cook until heated through and the marinara sauce is mostly evaporated.
4. Prepare the bell peppers by covering the two halves with the remaining olive oil (optional to also sprinkle with salt and pepper to taste).
5. Stuff each bell pepper with the meat and vegetable mixture. Transfer the bell peppers to a baking sheet and bake in the oven for 15 minutes.
6. Remove the baking sheet from the oven and top each bell pepper with 2 TBSP marinara sauce and 1 TBSP Parmesan cheese.
7. Return to the oven for an additional 8-10 minutes or until the cheese is melted and bell pepper is soft.

Nutrition Facts (1/2 of recipe):
258 calories, 19.5g protein, 21.5g carbohydrates, 11g fat

TIPS/SUGGESTIONS:
- Serve with a side salad or additional roasted vegetables for a yummy balanced meal.

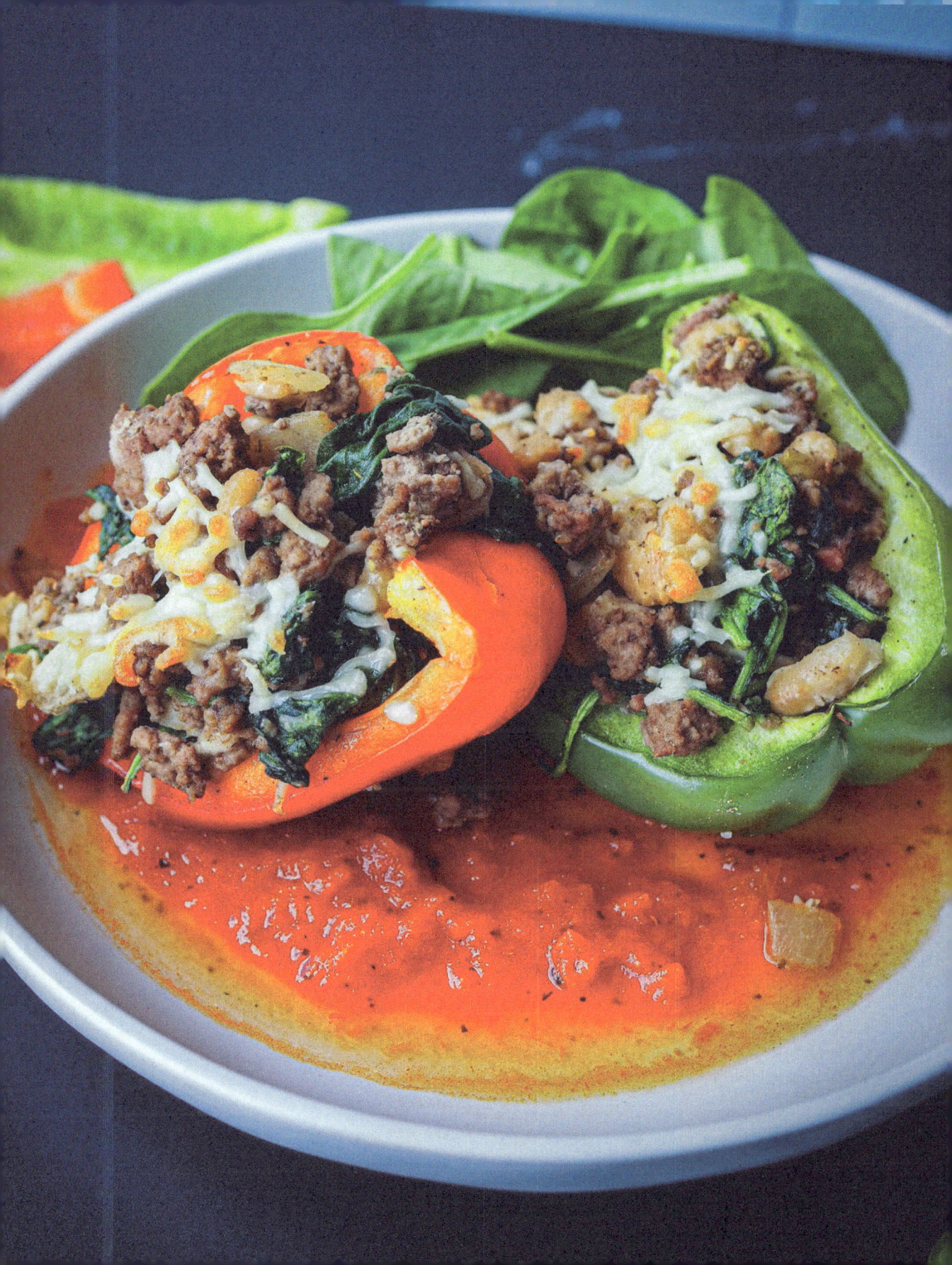

Part Seven: Dinner
BACON SWISS TURKEY BURGER

SERVINGS: 5 **MAKES: 5-6 BURGERS** **TIME: 30 MINUTES**

INGREDIENTS:

1 tsp olive oil
3 slices turkey bacon, diced
1/2 pound ground turkey
1/4 cup red onion, diced
4 cloves garlic, minced
1 TBSP almond flour
1/2 TBSP Worcestershire sauce
1/4 tsp salt
1/4 tsp pepper
1/4 tsp dried thyme
2-3 slices Swiss cheese

Optional ingredients:
Avocado
Slider bun
Pickles
Lettuce
Tomato

DIRECTIONS:

1. Preheat olive oil in a large pan over medium heat on the stove top.
2. Add turkey bacon to the pan and cook until crispy. Transfer bacon to a small plate and set aside. Return the pan to the stove top over medium heat.
3. In a medium-sized mixing bowl combine ground turkey, turkey bacon, red onion, garlic, almond flour, Worcestershire sauce, salt, pepper, and thyme. Using a wooden spoon (or your hands!), mix the ingredients together until well combined. Make sure to wash your hands well under hot water after touching raw poultry.
4. Measure about 2.5 ounces of the mixture, roll into a ball and flatten to create a burger. This recipe makes about five to six 2.5-ounce burgers. After forming the burgers place them in the preheated pan and allow to cook for about 8-10 minutes per side or until the internal temperature of each burger reaches 165 degrees F.
5. Top each burger with 1/2 slice Swiss cheese and include your favorite toppings!

● **GENERAL DIET**

Nutrition Facts (2.5-ounce burger):
153 calories, 14g protein, 3g carbohydrates, 10.5g fat

TIPS/SUGGESTIONS:
- You can serve this burger with a slider bun or have it over leafy greens with a low calorie salad dressing.

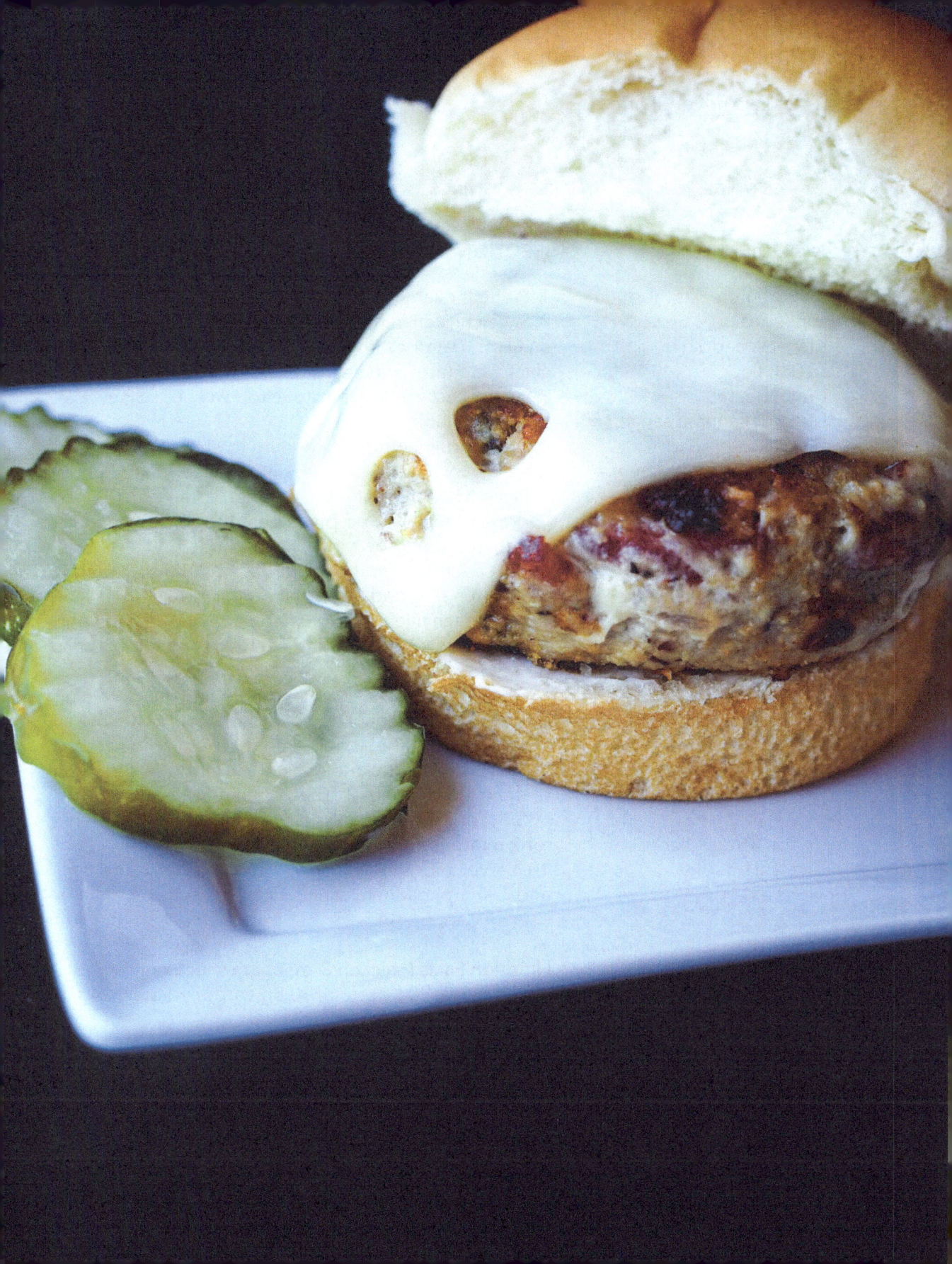

Part Seven: Dinner

CHICKEN PARMESAN

SERVINGS: 4 **MAKES: 4 SERVINGS** **TIME: 40 MINUTES**

INGREDIENTS:

2 chicken breasts (about 6 ounces each)
1 tsp avocado oil
2 TBSP flour
1 egg, beaten
1/2 cup marinara sauce, heated
4 TBSP mozzarella cheese
4 TBSP Parmesan cheese

Breading Ingredients:
2 TBSP almond flour
2 TBSP pine nuts
2 TBSP bread crumbs
1/4 cup Parmesan cheese
1/2 tsp salt
1/2 tsp pepper
1 tsp garlic powder
1/4 tsp dried thyme
1/2 tsp dried sage
1/4 tsp dried basil

Optional ingredients:
Zucchini noodles

● GENERAL DIET

DIRECTIONS:

1. Preheat oven to 400 degrees F.
2. Slice chicken in half lengthwise, making 4 thin chicken fillets, pat dry with a paper towel, salt, and pepper chicken to taste and set aside.
3. Heat a cast iron on the stove top with 1 TBSP avocado oil on medium heat.
4. Breading: Include all breading ingredients into a food processor and process until well combined.
5. Place three plates on the counter, sprinkle 2 TBSP of flour on one plate, and place beaten egg on one plate and the breading on the last plate.
6. Take each chicken fillet and dust with flour. Dip into the beaten egg and then coat with crust.
7. Place each fillet in the cast iron and cook for 4-5 minutes on each side, browning each side to create a crisp breading.
8. Once each side is crispy and browned, place the cast iron in preheated oven for 8-10 minutes, or until the internal temperature of chicken reaches 165 degrees F.
9. Once chicken is done cooking, take the cast iron out of the oven, top with 2 TBSP mozzarella cheese and 1 TBSP Parmesan cheese and place back into the oven for 2 minutes.
10. Serve chicken over 1/4-1/2 cup zucchini noodles and 1/4 cup marinara sauce. Enjoy!

Nutrition Facts (chicken & marinara sauce only):
297 calories, 30g protein, 10.5g carbohydrates, 14g fat

TIPS/SUGGESTIONS:
- Set up and measure out ingredients before starting the recipe to make for an easier assembly of the chicken.
- Make sure to wash your hands well with hot water after handling raw poultry.

MEATLOAF

SERVINGS: 8-10   **MAKES: 1 LARGE LOAF**   **TIME: 1 HOUR 15 MINUTES**

INGREDIENTS:

For the meatloaf:
- 1 pound lean ground beef
- 1 small white onion, minced
- 1/2 zucchini, shredded
- 1 egg
- 1/2 cup bread crumbs
- 1/4 cup Parmesan cheese
- 1/4 cup 1% milk
- 1 TBSP Worcestershire sauce
- 1/2 tsp Italian seasoning
- 1 tsp salt
- 1/2 tsp pepper
- 4-5 cloves garlic, minced
- 1 TBSP Dijon mustard
- 1 TBSP tomato paste

For the glaze:
- 2 TBSP tomato paste
- 2 tsp brown sugar
- 2 tsp apple cider vinegar
- 1/4 cup ketchup

DIRECTIONS:

1. Preheat oven to 400 degrees F and line a loaf pan with parchment paper or spray with oil.
2. After using cheese shredder to shred the zucchini, wrap in a paper towel and squeeze the excess liquid out.
3. Combine all meatloaf ingredients in a large bowl and mix with a wooden spoon or your hands until well combined.
4. Transfer the meatloaf mixture into the loaf pan, and using your hands press into the loaf pan to form the meatloaf (pack it in well and press down firmly).
5. Put the loaf pan into the oven and bake for 45 minutes. While the meatloaf is baking, prepare the glaze: combine all glaze ingredients in a small bowl and whisk with a fork until it's well combined.
6. Once the meatloaf is done cooking, remove from the oven and brush the glaze over the top. Return to the oven for another 15 minutes.
7. Remove from the oven and let the meatloaf cool for about 5 minutes before serving.

● **GENERAL DIET**

Nutrition Facts (1/8 of loaf):
165 calories, 14g protein, 11g carbohydrates, 6g fat

TIPS/SUGGESTIONS:
- Make sure to wash your hands well under hot water after handling raw meat.
- Serve with a side salad, mashed cauliflower, or roasted vegetables.

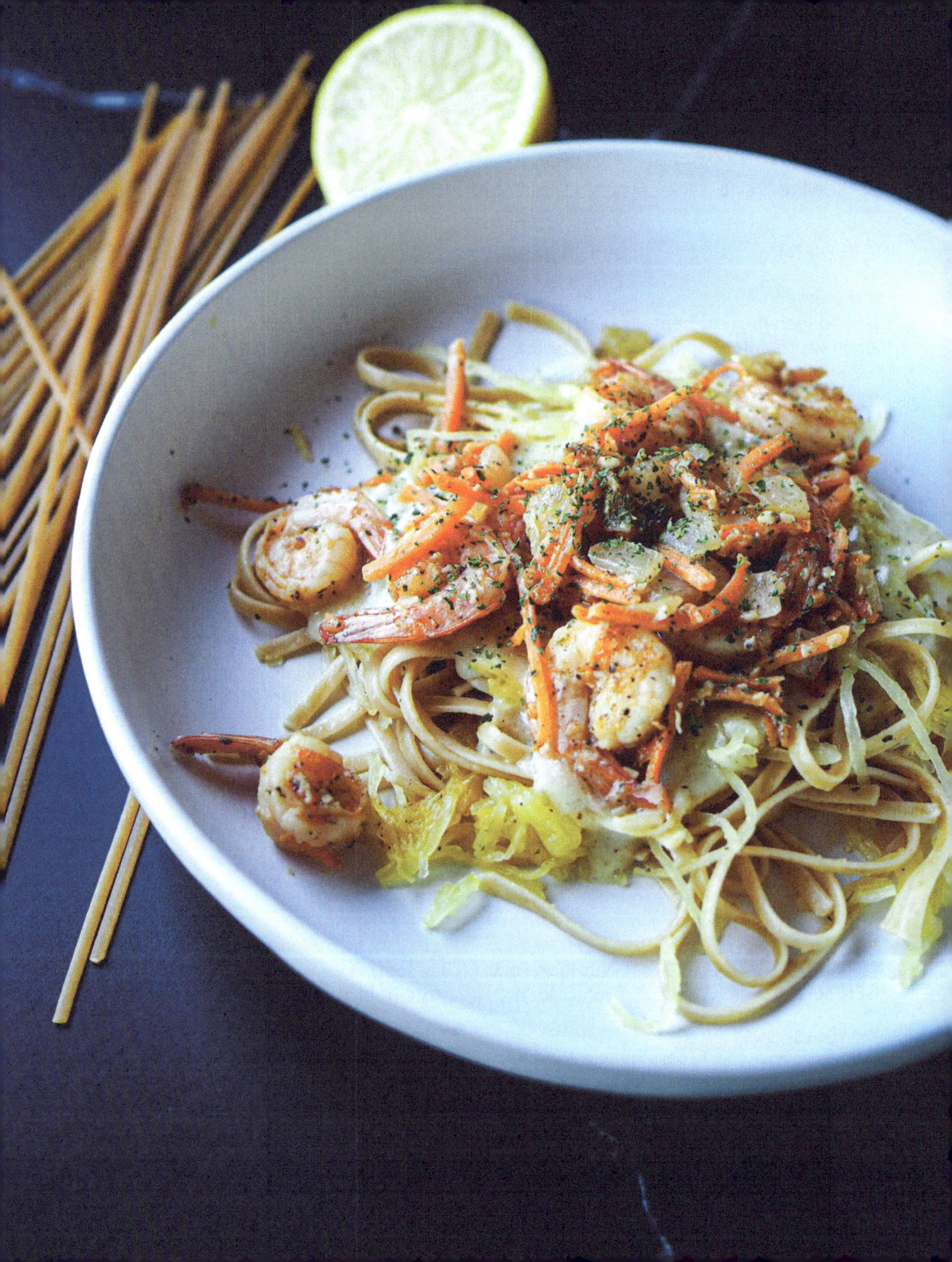

PARMESAN SHRIMP LINGUINE

SERVINGS: 5 **MAKES: ABOUT 5 CUPS** **TIME: 50 MINUTES**

INGREDIENTS:

- 1 spaghetti squash, halved lengthwise and seeds removed
- 3 tsp olive oil, divided
- Salt/pepper
- 2 TBSP butter
- 2 TBSP flour
- 1 cup chicken broth
- 1/2 cup 1% milk
- 1/2 tsp garlic powder
- 1/4 cup shredded Parmesan cheese
- 1/4 cup shredded asiago cheese
- 1/4 cup onion, diced
- 1/2 cup shredded carrots
- 3-4 cloves garlic, minced
- 3/4 pound shrimp
- 1/4 cup white wine (optional)
- Juice of 1/2 lemon
- 1 1/4 cup linguine, cooked

● GENERAL DIET

DIRECTIONS:

1. Preheat oven to 400 degrees F.
2. Prepare the spaghetti squash: Rub each squash half with 1 tsp olive oil and salt/pepper to taste. Lay face-down on a baking sheet and prick holes throughout the tops with a fork. Bake in the oven for 30-40 minutes. Once the squash is done baking, remove from the oven, allow to cool, then shred with a fork.
3. While the squash is baking, prepare the sauce: Preheat a small pot over low-medium heat on the stove top. Melt butter in the pan then sprinkle with flour. Whisk together, this should create a thickened mixture. Pour in broth and milk, whisking constantly until smooth. Bring to a low boil and add 1/2 tsp salt, 1/4 tsp pepper, and garlic powder. Then add Parmesan cheese and asiago cheese; stir until cheeses melt and sauce is thick and creamy. Cover and set aside.
4. Prepare the shrimp: Preheat 1 tsp olive oil in a large pan over medium-high heat. Add the onion, carrots, and garlic. Stir until fragrant, about 3-4 minutes. Add shrimp to the pan and season with salt and pepper to taste. Pour in white wine and lemon juice; let the mixture cook for about 8 minutes or until the shrimps are cooked through and the liquid has evaporated.
5. To portion, layer 1/4 cup linguine, 1/4 cup spaghetti squash, 1/4 cup sauce, and 1/4-1/2 cup of shrimp and vegetable mixture. Sprinkle with parsley and lemon juice if you want!

Nutrition Facts (as portioned in step #5):
263 calories, 20g protein, 19g carbohydrates, 12g fat

TIPS/SUGGESTIONS:
- If you are unable to tolerate pasta or are looking for a lower carb option, simply use spaghetti squash and don't include the linguine.

Part Seven: Dinner

CHICKEN FAJITA LETTUCE WRAPS

SERVINGS: 3 **MAKES: 3 FAJITAS** **TIME: 25 MINUTES**

INGREDIENTS:

1 TBSP olive oil, divided
1 large boneless, skinless chicken breast (about 6-9 ounces)
1/4 tsp salt, divided
1/4 tsp pepper, divided
1 tsp chili powder
1 tsp garlic powder
1/2 tsp cumin
1/2 large carrot, peeled
1/4 green bell pepper, sliced
1/4 red bell pepper, sliced
1/8 onion, sliced
Lettuce wrap or tortilla

Optional toppings:
Sour cream
Avocado
Hot sauce
Salsa

DIRECTIONS:

1. Preheat 1/2 TBSP olive oil in a large pan over medium-high heat on the stove top.
2. While the pan is preheating, slice the chicken lengthwise into small strips and slice the carrot lengthwise into matchsticks.
3. Place chicken into the pan, season with 1/8 tsp salt, 1/8 tsp pepper, chili powder, garlic powder, and cumin. Toss to coat the chicken evenly with the seasoning. Cook on the stove top for 10-12 minutes or until the chicken reaches an internal temperature of 165 degrees F, flipping the chicken every couple of minutes.
4. Once the chicken is cooked through, transfer to a small plate and set aside.
5. Using the same pan, preheat 1/2 TBSP olive oil over medium-high heat.
6. Place the carrots, bell peppers, and onion into the pan. Season with 1/8 tsp salt and 1/8 tsp pepper, let the vegetables cook for 8-10 minutes or until softened, flipping the vegetables every couple of minutes.
7. Assemble your fajita into a lettuce wrap or a low carb tortilla with chicken, cooked vegetables and any additional toppings. These fajitas are also great as lunch leftovers!

● GENERAL DIET

Nutrition Facts (1/3 of recipe without optional toppings):
160 calories, 13g protein, 2g carbohydrates, 11g fat

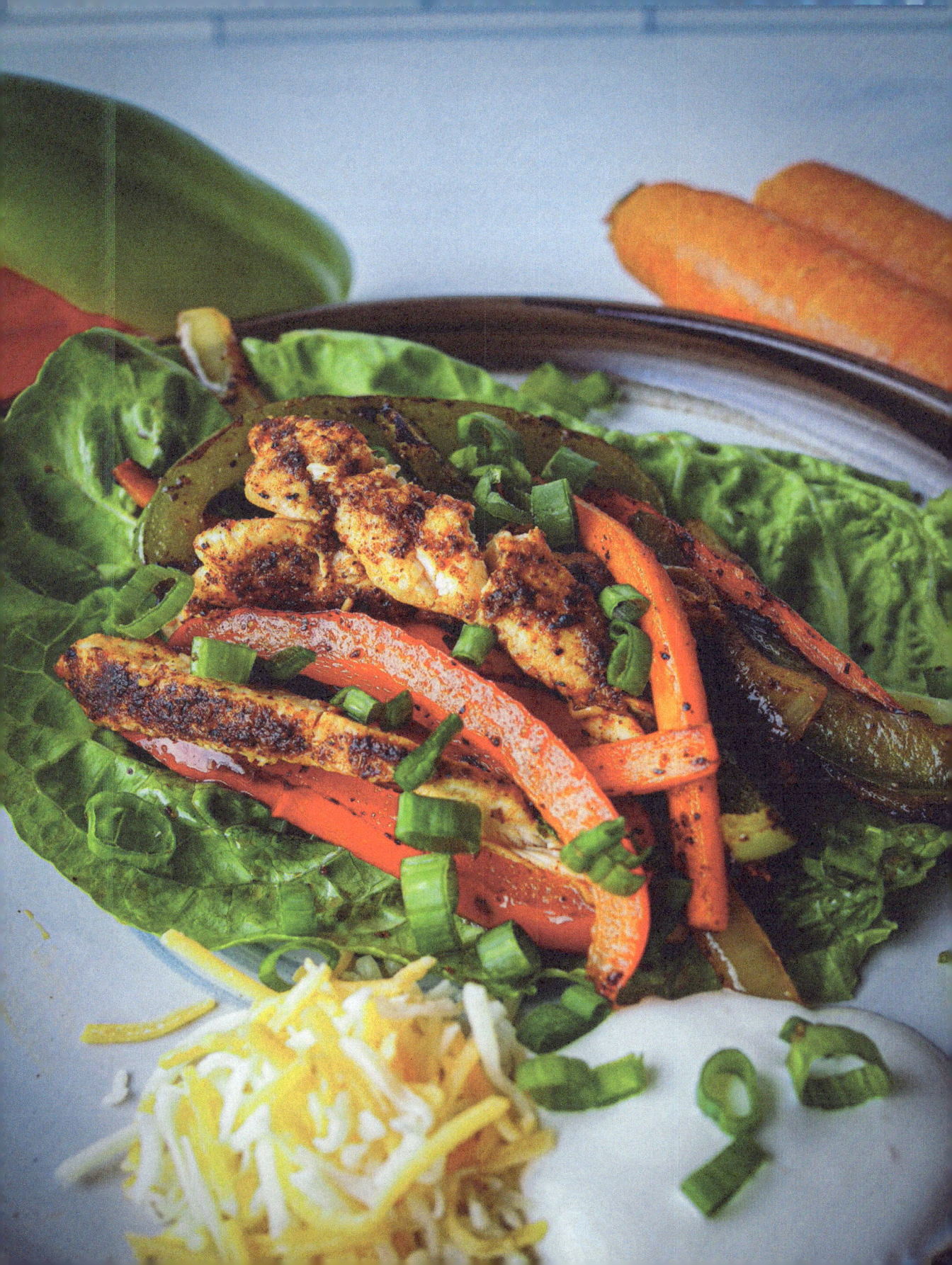

Part Eight: Snacks

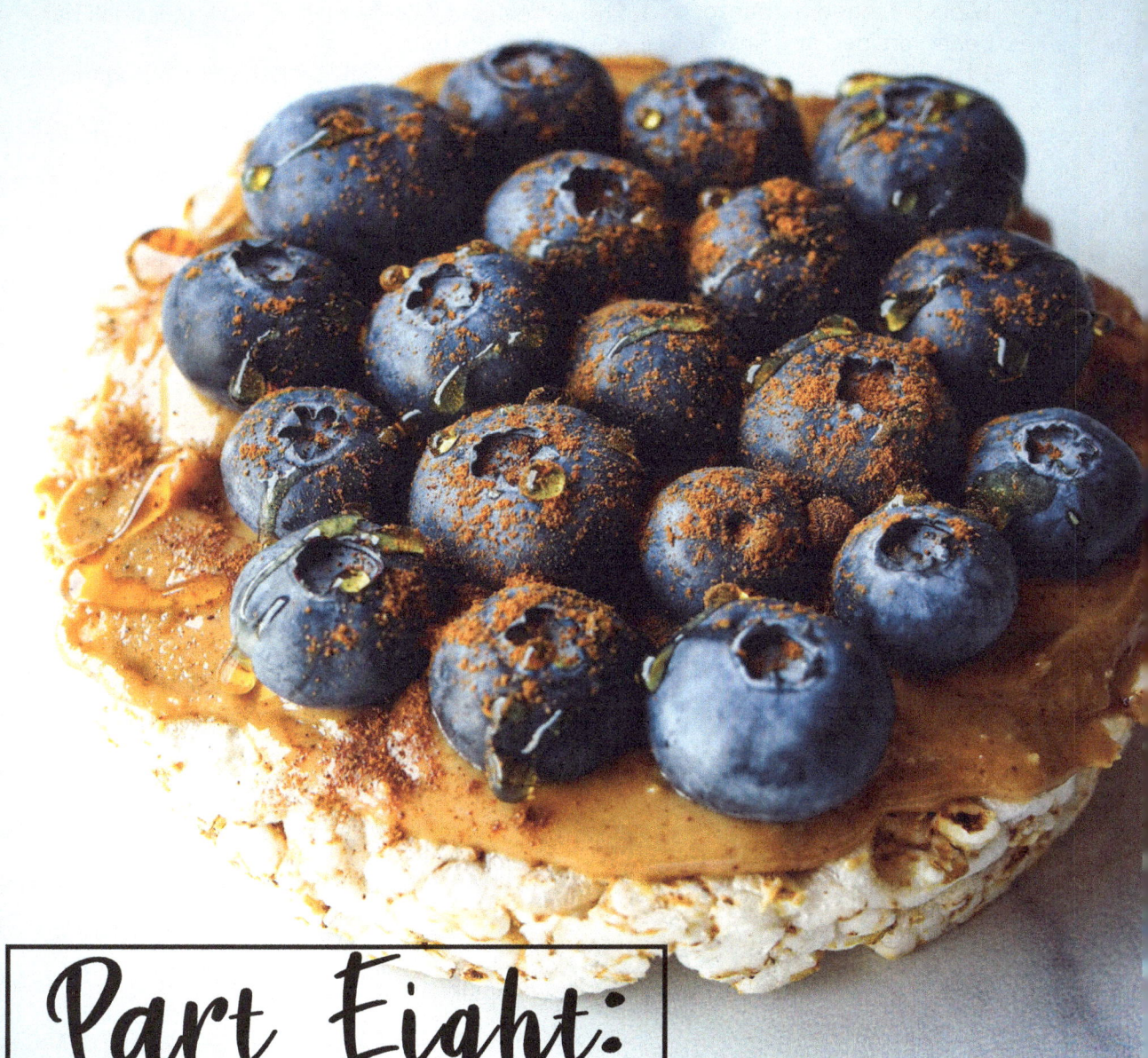

Part Eight:
SNACKS

ROASTED CHICKPEAS

INGREDIENTS:

1/2 cup canned garbanzo beans, drained and rinsed
1 tsp olive oil
1/8 tsp salt
1/8 tsp pepper
1/4 tsp garlic powder
1/8 tsp paprika

DIRECTIONS:

1. Preheat oven to 425 degrees F and line a small baking sheet with tin foil.
2. Toss garbanzo beans, olive oil, salt, pepper, garlic powder, and paprika in a small bowl.
3. Spread out garbanzo beans onto the baking sheet into a single layer.
4. Place baking sheet in the oven and bake for 8 minutes. Take baking sheet out of the oven, toss the garbanzo beans with a spatula, and return to the oven for another 8-10 minutes.

Nutrition Facts:
160 calories, 7g protein, 21g carbohydrates, 6g fat

AVOCADO FETA & EGG SALAD

INGREDIENTS:

1/4 avocado, diced
1 TBSP feta cheese, crumbled
1 hardboiled egg, diced
Salt/pepper, to taste
1 TBSP lemon juice

DIRECTIONS:

1. Mix together all ingredients in a small bowl. Enjoy!

Nutrition Facts:
184 calories, 8g protein, 4g carbohydrates, 14g fat

RICOTTA CRISP

INGREDIENTS:

1 multi-grain crispbread
2 TBSP ricotta cheese
1/2 TBSP basil pesto
4-5 slices cucumber
Pinch of salt/pepper

DIRECTIONS:

1. Spread ricotta cheese and basil pesto over crisp bread.
2. Sprinkle with salt and pepper, top with cucumber slices, and enjoy!

Nutrition Facts:
133 calories, 6.5g protein, 11g carbohydrates, 1.5g fat

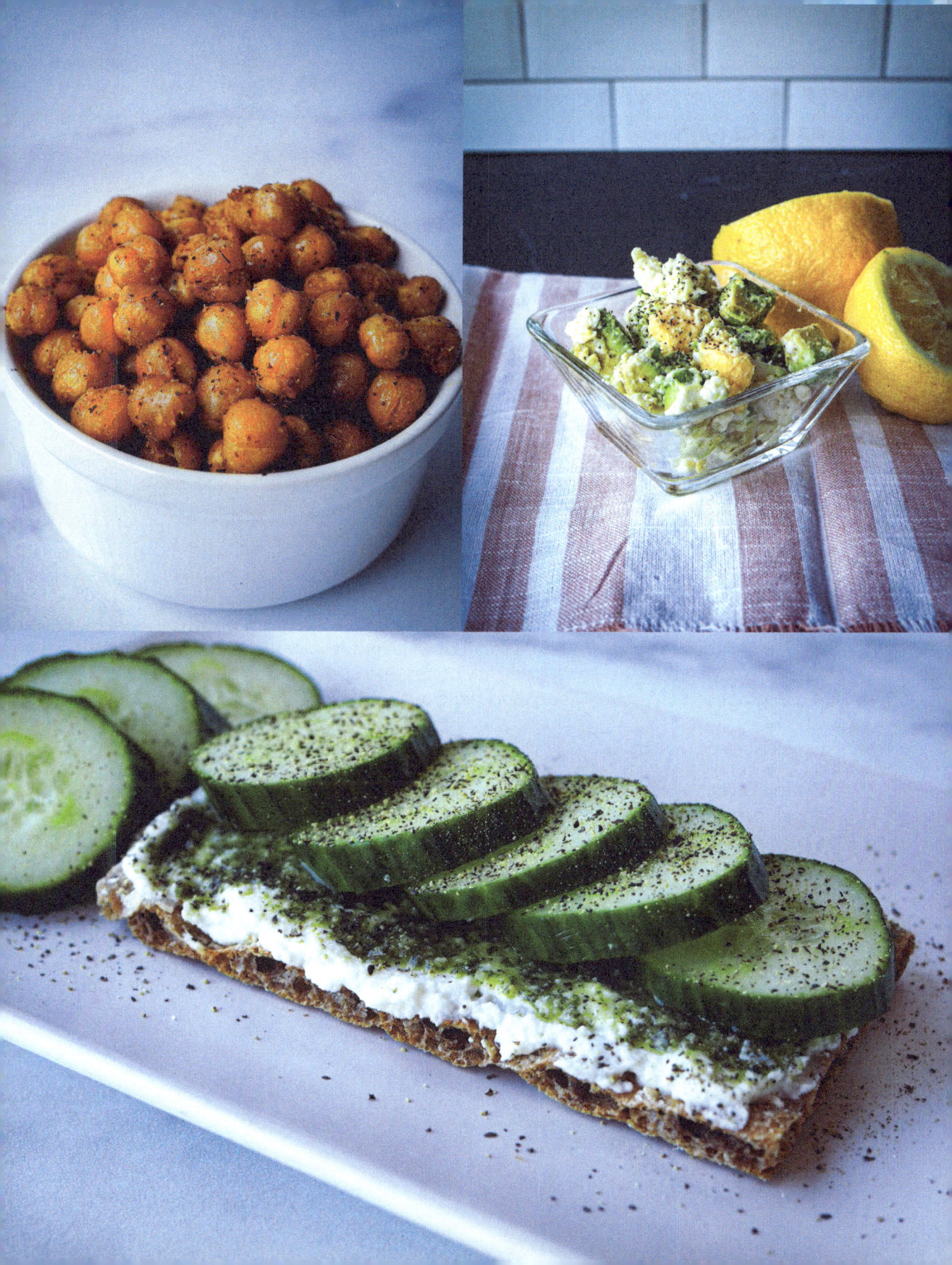

GREEK SALAD

INGREDIENTS:

2 TBSP diced cucumbers
2 TBSP diced red onion
2 TBSP canned chickpeas, drained and rinsed
2 TBSP black olives, sliced
2 slices deli turkey meat, chopped
1 TBSP low calorie Greek dressing or Italian dressing
1 TBSP feta cheese, crumbled

DIRECTIONS:

1. Combine cucumber, red onion, chickpeas, black olives, and turkey meat in a small bowl.
2. When ready to eat, drizzle with salad dressing and sprinkle with feta cheese.
3. Salt and pepper to taste, if you would like.
4. Prepare ahead of time: prep vegetables and portion into small containers. Don't drizzle with dressing or add cheese until you are ready to eat though!

Nutrition Facts:
145 calories, 12g protein, 8g carbohydrates, 7.5g fat

COTTAGE CHEESE & GRAPES

INGREDIENTS:

1/2 cup low fat cottage cheese
1/4 cup grapes
1 tsp honey
1 tsp chia seeds

DIRECTIONS:

1. In a small bowl layer the cottage cheese and grapes, drizzle with honey and sprinkle with chia seeds. Very easy and delicious!

Nutrition Facts:
152 calories, 14g protein, 16g carbohydrates, 3.5g fat

PARFAIT

INGREDIENTS:

1/4 cup low fat Greek yogurt (flavor of choice)
1/4 cup berries
2 TBSP granola

DIRECTIONS:

1. In a small bowl layer the Greek yogurt, berries, and the granola. If you want to add a little something extra sprinkle with cinnamon or drizzle with a small amount (no more than 1 tsp) of honey or pure maple syrup.

Nutrition Facts:
121 calories, 7g protein, 15.5g carbohydrates, 3g fat

HOMEMADE TRAIL MIX

INGREDIENTS:

1 cup whole raw almonds
1 cup cashews
1/4 cup pepitas
1/4 cup raisins or dried blueberries
1/4 cup dark chocolate chips

DIRECTIONS:

1. Combine all ingredients in a medium bowl.
2. Portion out into 1/4 cup servings into small bags or containers, and you will have a great go-to snack during the work week!

This recipe makes about 10 servings of trail mix.

Nutrition Facts (per 1/4 cup):
214 calories, 5.5g protein, 15g carbohydrates, 15g fat

APPLE OR PEAR + FRUIT DIP

INGREDIENTS:

1/2 apple or pear
5.3 ounces coconut flavored low fat Greek yogurt
1 TBSP peanut butter
1/8 tsp cinnamon

DIRECTIONS:

1. In a small bowl (or even straight into the yogurt cup) combine the yogurt, peanut butter and cinnamon.
3. Slice up the fruit and enjoy your dip.

Nutrition Facts:
232 calories, 16g protein, 21.5g carbohydrates, 10g fat

SPICY COTTAGE CHEESE + VEGGIES

INGREDIENTS:

1/2 cup low fat cottage cheese
1/2 TBSP favorite hot sauce
3 celery sticks
3 bell pepper sticks

DIRECTIONS:

1. In a small bowl, mix together the cottage cheese and hot sauce.
2. If you want to add something extra, you can include garlic powder, onion powder, salt, pepper, paprika, etc. Dip your veggies and enjoy.

Nutrition Facts:
111 calories, 14g protein, 9.5g carbohydrates, 2g fat

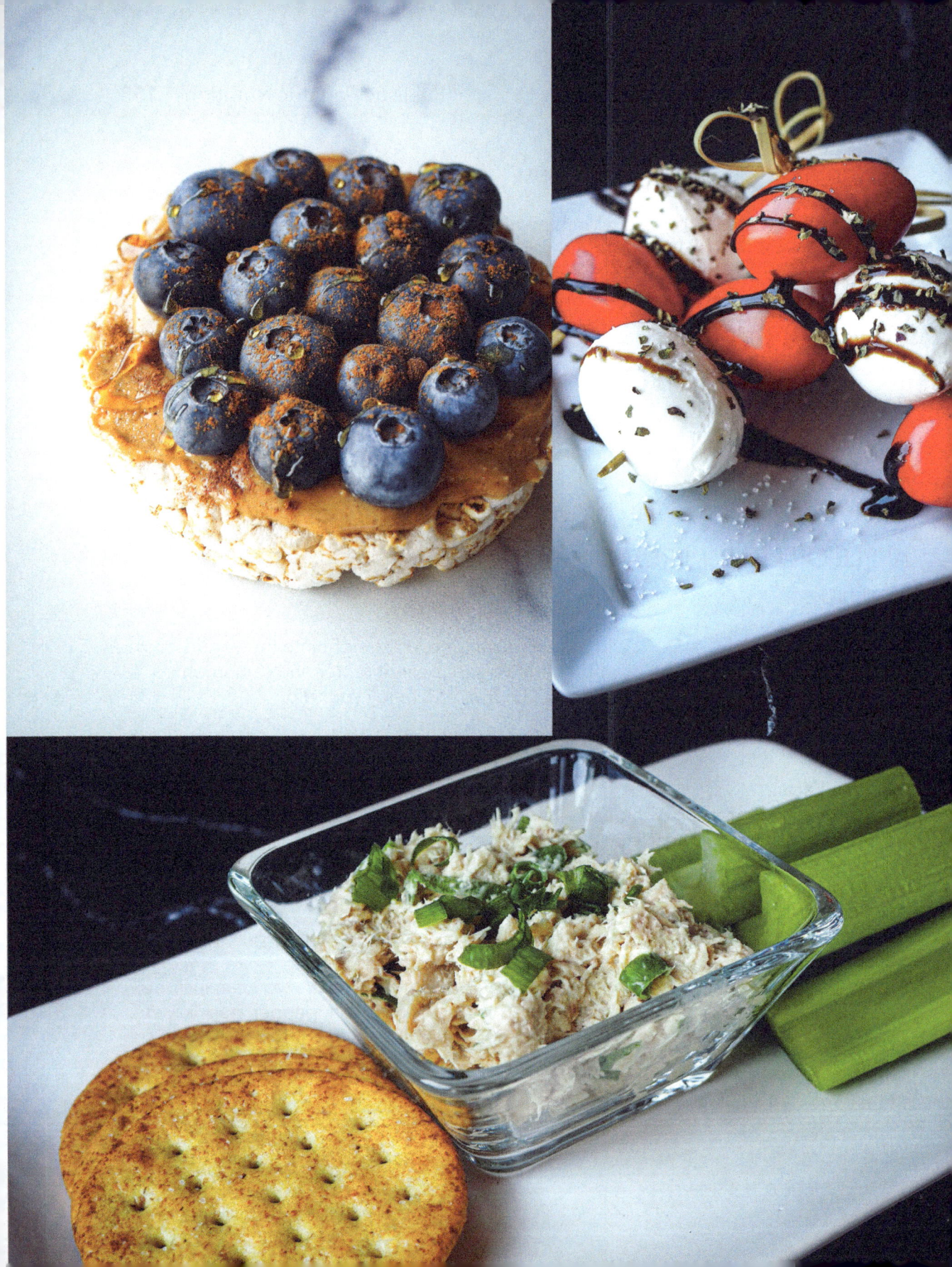

TUNA DIP

INGREDIENTS:

1 5-ounce can of tuna
1 TBSP cream cheese
1 tsp Dijon mustard
Salt/pepper to taste
3 whole wheat crackers
3-4 celery sticks

Optional ingredient:
1 TBSP green onions, sliced

DIRECTIONS:

1. In a small bowl, combine tuna, cream cheese, and mustard and mix well. Season with salt and pepper as you wish. If you are using green onions, mix these in with the tuna as well.
2. Serve with whole wheat crackers and celery sticks.

Nutrition Facts:
214 calories, 23g protein, 12.5g carbohydrates, 7.5g fat

BALSAMIC TOMATOES & MOZZARELLA

INGREDIENTS:

4 mozzarella balls
4 cherry tomatoes
1/2 TBSP balsamic glaze
Salt, to taste
1/4 tsp dried basil

DIRECTIONS:

1. You can either combine ingredients in a small bowl or use toothpicks to spear the tomatoes and mozzarella, then drizzle with balsamic glaze and sprinkle with salt and dried basil.

Nutrition Facts:
183 calories, 10.5g protein, 9.5g carbohydrates, 10g fat

BLUEBERRY RICE CAKE

INGREDIENTS:

1 lightly salted rice cake
2 TBSP peanut butter
1/4 cup fresh blueberries
1 tsp honey
Sprinkle of cinnamon

DIRECTIONS:

1. Spread the peanut butter over the rice cake in an even layer.
2. Arrange the blueberries in a single layer over the rice cake. Sprinkle with cinnamon and drizzle with honey.

Nutrition Facts:
265 calories, 8g protein, 24g carbohydrates, 16g fat

TEX-MEX SNACK

INGREDIENTS:

2 TBSP canned corn
2 TBSP black beans
2 ounces canned chicken, drained
Salt/pepper, to taste
1/4 tsp cumin
1 TBSP salsa
1/2 TBSP sour cream

DIRECTIONS:

1. In a small bowl, mix together corn, black beans, chicken, salt, pepper, and cumin.
2. When ready to eat, mix in the salsa and sour cream.
3. Make sure not to mix in the salsa and sour cream until you are ready to eat. Prep this snack ahead of time by making 3-4 of these in containers, then you have a ready made snack during the work week.

Nutrition Facts:
134 calories, 15.5g protein, 11g carbohydrates, 2.5g fat

MEAT AND HUMMUS ROLL UPS

INGREDIENTS:

2-3 slices deli meat of choice
2 TBSP hummus
1 TBSP Dijon mustard
3-4 veggie sticks (carrots, bell pepper, celery, pickle, etc)

DIRECTIONS:

1. Spread 1/3 of hummus and Dijon mustard over each slice of deli meat.
2. Place veggie sticks over top of each deli slice and roll up.

Nutrition Facts:
125 calories, 11.5g protein, 8g carbohydrates, 4g fat

BERRY SALAD

INGREDIENTS:

1/2 cup mixed berries
2 TBSP slivered almonds
2 TBSP pepitas
1 tsp honey
1 TBSP unsweetened shredded coconut

DIRECTIONS:

1. Mix all ingredients in a small bowl and enjoy! If you want to prepare this ahead of time for the work week, then wait until you are ready to eat before drizzling with honey.

Nutrition Facts:
222 calories, 5g protein, 24g carbohydrates, 12g fat

Meal Plans

2-4 MONTHS POST-SURGERY
158

4-6 MONTHS POST-SURGERY
162

6-12 MONTHS POST-SURGERY
166

12+ MONTHS POST-SURGERY
170

2-4 MONTHS POST-SURGERY

DAY #1	MEAL	CALORIES PROTEIN
BREAKFAST	5.3 ounces Greek yogurt 1/4 cup strawberries	101 calories 12g protein
LUNCH	1/2 buffalo chicken chaffle pg. 105	151 calories 17g protein
SNACK	Tropical sunrise protein shake pg. 36	201 calories 21g protein
DINNER	2 turkey and veggie meatballs pg. 120	172 calories 20g protein
		TOTAL: 625 calories 70g protein
DAY #2		
BREAKFAST	Strawberry banana smoothie pg. 62	198 calories 15g protein
LUNCH	1/2 buffalo chicken chaffle pg. 105	151 calories 17g protein
SNACK	Cottage cheese + grapes pg. 152	152 calories 14g protein
DINNER	1 roasted chicken thigh + 1/4 cup roasted veg	256 calories 28g protein
		TOTAL: 757 calories 74g protein

2-4 MONTHS POST-SURGERY

DAY #3	MEAL	CALORIES PROTEIN
BREAKFAST	Pre-made protein shake	160 calories 30g protein
LUNCH	1 chicken thigh + 1/4 cup roasted veg	256 calories 28g protein
SNACK	1/2 tuna dip recipe pg. 155	107 calories 11.5g protein
DINNER	2 turkey and veggie meatballs pg. 120	172 calories 20g protein
		TOTAL: 695 calories 89.5g protein
DAY #4		
BREAKFAST	2 protein bombs pg. 68	244 calories 13g protein
LUNCH	1/2 tuna dip recipe pg. 155	107 calories 11.5g protein
SNACK	3 slices deli meat + 1 pickle	75 calories 16.5g protein
DINNER	1/2 cup chicken tortilla soup pg. 100	141 calories 14g protein
SNACK	1 protein bomb pg. 68	122 calories 6.5g protein
		TOTAL: 689 calories 61.5g protein

Meal Plans

2-4 MONTHS POST-SURGERY

DAY #5	MEAL	CALORIES PROTEIN
BREAKFAST	Tropical sunrise protein shake pg. 36	201 calories 21g protein
LUNCH	Meat and vegetable rice cake pg. 101	153 calories 12g protein
SNACK	Pre-made protein shake	160 calories 30g protein
DINNER	1/2 cup chicken tortilla soup pg. 100	141 calories 14g protein
		TOTAL: 655 calories 77g protein
DAY #6		
BREAKFAST	Peanut butter banana smoothie pg. 61	266 calories 20.5g protein
LUNCH	1/2 cup chicken tortilla soup pg. 100	141 calories 14g protein
SNACK	5.3 ounces Greek yogurt 1/4 cup strawberries	101 calories 12g protein
DINNER	1 chicken fajita lettuce wrap pg. 146	160 calories 13g protein
SNACK	2 slices deli meat + 1 pickle	55 calories 11g protein
		TOTAL: 723 calories 70.5g protein

2-4 MONTHS POST-SURGERY

DAY #7	MEAL	CALORIES PROTEIN
BREAKFAST	2 protein bombs pg. 68	244 calories 13g protein
LUNCH	Pre-made protein shake	160 calories 30g protein
SNACK	Meat and vegetable rice cake pg. 101	153 calories 12g protein
DINNER	1 chicken fajita lettuce wrap pg. 146	160 calories 13g protein
		TOTAL: 717 calories 68g protein

4-6 MONTHS POST-SURGERY

DAY #1	MEAL	CALORIES PROTEIN
BREAKFAST	Pre-made protein shake	160 calories 30g protein
LUNCH	Tex-Mex snack pg. 156	134 calories 15.5g protein
SNACK	Blueberry rice cake pg. 155	265 calories 8g protein
DINNER	3 ounces ground beef + 1/2 cup marinara + zucchini noodles	229 calories 20g protein
		TOTAL: 778 calories 73.5g protein
DAY #2		
BREAKFAST	1 tomato basil omelette pg. 77	138 calories 10g protein
SNACK	Avocado, feta, and egg salad pg. 150	184 calories 8g protein
LUNCH	Curry chickpea soup + 1/4-1/2 cup salad pg. 45	201 calories 24g protein
SNACK	1 string cheese + 1/2 apple	148 calories 7g protein
DINNER	3 ounces ground beef + 1/2 cup marinara + zucchini noodles	229 calories 20g protein
		TOTAL: 900 calories 96g protein

Realistic Bariatric Nutrition | 163

4-6 MONTHS POST-SURGERY

DAY #3	MEAL	CALORIES PROTEIN
BREAKFAST	Blueberry rice cake pg. 155	265 calories 8g protein
LUNCH	Curry chickpea soup + 1/4-1/2 cup salad pg. 45	201 calories 24g protein
SNACK	5.3 ounces Greek yogurt + 1/2 apple	138 calories 12g protein
DINNER	Parmesan shrimp linguine pg. 145	263 calories 20g protein
		TOTAL: 867 calories 64g protein
DAY #4		
BREAKFAST	Lemon blueberry protein shake pg. 33	151 calories 21g protein
LUNCH	Curry chickpea soup + 1/4-1/2 cup salad pg. 45	201 calories 24g protein
SNACK	Berry salad pg. 156	222 calories 5g protein
DINNER	Parmesan shrimp linguine pg. 145	263 calories 64g protein
		TOTAL: 837 calories 70g protein

4-6 MONTHS POST-SURGERY

DAY #5	MEAL	CALORIES PROTEIN
BREAKFAST	Pre-made protein shake	160 calories 30g protein
LUNCH	1 cobb salad pg. 82	174 calories 12g protein
SNACK	Apple or pear + fruit dip pg. 153	232 calories 16g protein
DINNER	1 chicken burger + 1/4 cup roasted vegetables pg. 124	190 calories 13g protein
		TOTAL: 756 calories 71g protein
DAY #6		
BREAKFAST	Sweet potato vegetable hash pg. 64	219 calories 13g protein
SNACK	1/2 wild berry smoothie pg. 60	104 calories 13g protein
LUNCH	1 cobb salad pg. 82	174 calories 12g protein
SNACK	5.3 ounces Greek yogurt + 1 TBSP peanut butter	174 calories 16g protein
DINNER	1 chicken burger + 1/4 cup roasted vegetables pg. 124	190 calories 13g protein
		TOTAL: 861 calories 67g protein

4-6 MONTHS POST-SURGERY

DAY #7	MEAL	CALORIES PROTEIN
BREAKFAST	Sweet potato vegetable hash pg. 64	219 calories 13g protein
SNACK	1/2 wild berry smoothie pg. 60	104 calories 13g protein
LUNCH	1 chicken burger + 1/4 cup roasted vegetables pg. 124	190 calories 13g protein
SNACK	1 string cheese + 1/2 apple	148 calories 7g protein
DINNER	1 cup chicken and broccoli bake pg. 134	232 calories 28g protein
		TOTAL: 893 calories 74g protein

6-12 MONTHS POST-SURGERY

DAY #1	MEAL	CALORIES PROTEIN
BREAKFAST	5.3 ounces Greek yogurt + grain-free granola pg. 77	246 calories 16g protein
LUNCH	Taco salad pg. 103	281 calories 14g protein
SNACK	1/4 cup almonds + 2 slices deli meat	215 calories 17g protein
DINNER	Beef and bean jalapeno chili pg. 106	229 calories 19g protein
		TOTAL: 971 calories 66g protein
DAY #2		
BREAKFAST	Banana nut protein shake pg. 33	217 calories 30g protein
SNACK	String cheese	90 calories 7g protein
LUNCH	Beef and bean jalapeno chili pg. 106	229 calories 19g protein
SNACK	Spicy cottage cheese & veggies pg. 153	111 calories 14g protein
DINNER	Stuffed pork chop pg. 116	232 calories 18g protein
		TOTAL: 879 calories 88g protein

6-12 MONTHS POST-SURGERY

DAY #3	MEAL	CALORIES PROTEIN
BREAKFAST	Pre-made protein shake + 1/2 cup berries	202 calories 30g protein
LUNCH	Stuffed pork chop pg. 116	232 calories 18g protein
SNACK	Parfait pg. 152	121 calories 7g protein
DINNER	Chicken sausage & veggies pg. 137	284 calories 16g protein
		TOTAL: 839 calories 71g protein
DAY #4		
BREAKFAST	Loaded avocado toast pg. 70	241 calories 18g protein
LUNCH	Beef and bean jalapeno chili pg. 106	229 calories 19g protein
SNACK	Tuna dip pg. 155	214 calories 23g protein
DINNER	Chicken sausage & veggies pg. 137	284 calories 16g protein
		TOTAL: 968 calories 76g protein

6-12 MONTHS POST-SURGERY

DAY #5	MEAL	CALORIES PROTEIN
BREAKFAST	Blueberry pie smoothie pg. 62	235 calories 15g protein
LUNCH	Chicken sausage & veggies pg. 137	284 calories 16g protein
SNACK	Mocha protein shake pg. 32	233 calories 23g protein
DINNER	Turkey taco lettuce wrap pg. 114	144 calories 12g protein
		TOTAL: 896 calories 66g protein
DAY #6		
BREAKFAST	Mocha protein shake pg. 32	231 calories 31g protein
SNACK	1/2 pre-made protein shake + 1/2 banana	105 calories 15g protein
LUNCH	Turkey taco lettuce wrap pg. 114	144 calories 12g protein
SNACK	1/2 pre-made protein shake + 1/2 banana	105 calories 15g protein
DINNER	Jalapeno cheddar salmon cake + 1/4 cup roasted vegetables pg. 98	130 calories 9g protein
		TOTAL: 715 calories 82g protein

6-12 MONTHS POST-SURGERY

DAY #7	MEAL	CALORIES PROTEIN
BREAKFAST	Coconut dream protein shake pg. 35	229 calories 30g protein
SNACK	1 string cheese + 1/4 cup almonds	255 calories 13g protein
LUNCH	Jalapeno cheddar salmon cake + 1/4 cup roasted vegetables pg. 98	130 calories 9g protein
SNACK	5.3 ounces Greek yogurt + 1/2 cup strawberries	120 calories 12g protein
DINNER	Turkey & veg sandwich pg. 86	182 calories 17g protein
		TOTAL: 916 calories 81g protein

12+ MONTHS POST-SURGERY

DAY #1	MEAL	CALORIES PROTEIN
BREAKFAST	Pineapple mango smoothie + 1/2 scoop protein powder pg. 61	279 calories 23.5g protein
LUNCH	Apple pecan salad pg. 108	296 calories 16.5g protein
SNACK	4-5 celery sticks + 2 TBSP peanut butter	200 calories 8g protein
DINNER	Chicken enchiladas pg. 132	240 calories 16.5g protein
		TOTAL: 1015 calories 64.5g protein
DAY #2		
BREAKFAST	1/2 bacon cheddar chaffle + 1/2 apple pg. 74	217 calories 10.5g protein
LUNCH	Chicken enchiladas pg. 132	240 calories 16.5g protein
SNACK	5.3 ounces Greek yogurt + 1 TBSP peanut butter	177 calories 16g protein
DINNER	Beef and vegetable teriyaki pg. 122	328 calories 28g protein
		TOTAL: 962 calories 71g protein

Realistic Bariatric Nutrition

12+ MONTHS POST-SURGERY

DAY #3	MEAL	CALORIES PROTEIN
BREAKFAST	1/2 bacon cheddar chaffle + 1/2 apple pg. 74	217 calories 10.5g protein
LUNCH	Beef and vegetable teriyaki pg. 122	328 calories 28g protein
SNACK	Balsamic tomatoes & mozzarella pg. 155	183 calories 10.5g protein
DINNER	Coconut chicken curry + 1/4 cup brown rice pg. 126	224 calories 18g protein
		TOTAL: 952 calories 67g protein
DAY #4		
BREAKFAST	Pre-made protein shake + 1 banana	265 calories 30g protein
SNACK	4-5 celery sticks + 2 TBSP peanut butter	200 calories 8g protein
LUNCH	Coconut chicken curry + 1/4 cup brown rice pg. 126	224 calories 18g protein
SNACK	Roasted chickpeas + 1/2 cup grapes pg. 150	191 calories 7g protein
DINNER	Sausage and potato soup pg. 88	134 calories 13.5g protein
		TOTAL: 1014 calories 76.5g protein

12+ MONTHS POST-SURGERY

DAY #5	MEAL	CALORIES PROTEIN
BREAKFAST	Overnight oats pg. 72	306 calories 26g protein
LUNCH	Coconut chicken curry + 1/4 cup brown rice pg. 126	224 calories 18g protein
SNACK	5.3 ounces yogurt + grain-free granola pg. 79	246 calories 16g protein
DINNER	Sausage and potato soup + 1/2 cup salad pg. 88	179 calories 13.5g protein
		TOTAL: 955 calories 73.5g protein
DAY #6		
BREAKFAST	Green smoothie pg. 60	207 calories 13g protein
SNACK	Homemade trail mix pg. 153	214 calories 5.5g protein
LUNCH	Sausage and potato soup + 1/2 cup salad pg. 88	179 calories 13.5g protein
SNACK	Pre-made protein shake, 2 TBSP hummus + 5 baby carrots	230 calories 32g protein
DINNER	Burrito bowl pg. 125	212 calories 17g protein
		TOTAL: 1042 calories 81g protein

12+ MONTHS POST-SURGERY

DAY #7	MEAL	CALORIES PROTEIN
BREAKFAST	Orange cream protein shake pg. 32	225 calories 30g protein
LUNCH	Burrito bowl pg. 125	212 calories 17g protein
SNACK	Homemade trail mix pg. 153	214 calories 5.5g protein
DINNER	Herbed chicken + mashed cauli pg. 112	313 calories 30g protein
		TOTAL: 964 calories 82.5g protein

RESOURCES

AMERICAN SOCIETY FOR METABOLIC AND BARIATRIC SURGERY
https://asmbs.org

ACADEMY OF NUTRITION AND DIETETICS
https://www.eatright.org

BARIATRIC TIMES
https://bariatrictimes.com

OBESITY ACTION COALITION
https://www.obesityaction.org

INTERNATIONAL FEDERATION FOR THE SURGERY OF OBESITY AND METABOLIC DISORDERS (IFSO)
https://www.ifso.com

ACKNOWLEDGMENTS

Thank you to the following individuals for your help and input in creating this book:

Erica Anderl
Amanda Buschman
Jennifer Ramsrud RDN, CDCES
Cory Richardson MD, FACS, FASMBS

RECIPE INDEX

Apple
cinnamon oatmeal, 51
fruit dip, 153
peanut butter protein shake, 35
pecan salad, 108, *109*
pie protein shake, 34

Avocado
bacon swiss turkey burger, 140, *141*
beef and bean jalapeno chili, 106, *107*
burrito bowls, 125
chicken fajita lettuce wraps, 146, *147*
chicken tortilla soup, 100
cobb salad, 82, *83*
feta & egg salad, 150, *151*
green smoothie, 60
meat and vegetable rice cake, 101
one pan chicken sausage and veg, 137
sausage chaffle, 75
sweet potato vegetable hash, 64, *65*
toast, loaded, 70, *71*

Banana
chia seed pudding, 68
green smoothie, 60
nut protein shake, 33
peanut butter banana smoothie, 61
pineapple mango smoothie, 61
strawberry banana smoothie, 62
yogurt parfait, 50

Bean
and vegetable soup, 97
and walnut burgers, 92, *93*
beef & bean jalapeno chili, 106, *107*
black bean sweet potato tacos, 118
burrito bowls, 125
chicken burgers, 124
chickpea burger with caesar salad, 96
chickpea tuna salad, 84, *85*
chicken tortilla soup, 100
coconut chicken curry, 126, *127*
curry chickpea soup, *44*, 45
fiesta cauliflower rice, 90, *91*
roasted chickpeas, 150, *151*
sausage & veggie skillet, 129
southwest eggs, 50
spring thyme vegetable soup, 53
stuffed bell peppers, 138, *139*
tex-mex snack, 156
tortilla-less chicken enchiladas, 132, *133*
turkey tacos, 114, *115*
vegetable chili, 54
white bean chili verde, 55

Beef
and bean jalapeno chili, 106, *107*
and vegetable teriyaki, 122, *123*
meatloaf, 143
protein content, 19
shepherd's pie, 128
stuffed bell peppers, 138, *139*

Blueberry
pie, smoothie, 62
lemon blueberry protein shake, 33
rice cake, *149, 154*, 155

Burgers
bacon swiss turkey burger, 140, *141*
bean and walnut burger, 92, *93*
chicken burger, 124

Broccoli
beef and vegetable teriyaki, 122, *123*
cheddar soup, 56, *57*
chicken and broccoli bake, 134, *135*
one pan salmon and broccoli, 136
stuffed pork chops, 116, *117*

Cauliflower
asiago soup, 40, *41*
coconut chicken curry, 126, *127*
cream of asparagus soup, *39*, 43
curry chickpea soup, *44*, 45
herbed chicken with mashed cauli, 112, *113*

Recipe Index

Cauliflower (cont'd)
mashed cauliflower, 51
rice, fiesta, 90, *91*
sausage and potato soup, 88, *89*
shepherd's pie, 128
vegetable chili, 54

Chaffle
asparagus pesto chaffle, 104
bacon cheddar chaffle, 74
buffalo chicken chaffle, 105
garden vegetable chaffle, 101
sausage chaffle, 75

Cheddar
bacon cheddar chaffle, 74
broccoli cheddar soup, *56*, 57
chicken & broccoli bake, 134, *135*
jalapeno cheddar salmon cakes, 98, *99*

Chicken
and broccoli bake, 134, *135*
buffalo chicken chaffle, 105
burgers, 124
burrito bowls, 125
cobb salad, 82, *83*
coconut chicken curry 126, *127*
fajita lettuce wraps, 146, *147*
grape & walnut salad, 94, *95*
herbed chicken with mashed cauli, 112, *113*
loaded avocado toast, 70, *71*
one pan chicken sausage & vegetables, 137
parmesan, 142
protein content, 19
roasted vegetable pasta salad, *130*, 131
sausage and potato soup, 88, *89*
sweet potato vegetable hash, 64
tex-mex snack, 156
tortilla-less enchiladas, 132, *133*
tortilla soup, 100
white bean chili verde, 55

Chickpea
burger with caesar salad, 96
curry chickpea soup, *44*, 45

greek salad, 152
roasted chickpeas, 150, *151*
tuna salad, 84, *85*

Egg
asparagus pesto chaffle, 104
avocado feta & egg salad, 150, *151*
bacon cheddar chaffle, 74
buffalo chicken chaffle, 105
chicken parmesan, 142
chickpea burger with caesar salad, 96
cobb salad, 82, *83*
garden vegetable chaffle, 101
jalapeno cheddar salmon cakes, 98, *99*
meatloaf, 143
mediterranean frittata, 66, *67*
protein content, 19
sausage chaffle, 75
southwest eggs, 50
sweet potato vegetable hash, 64, *65*
tomato basil omelette, 76, *77*

Lettuce Wrap
chicken fajita lettuce wraps 146, *147*
chicken grape and walnut salad, 94, *95*
chickpea tuna salad, 84, *85*
turkey tacos, 114, *115*

Milk
apple cinnamon oatmeal, 51
broccoli cheddar soup, *56*, 57
chia seed pudding, 68
cream of asparagus soup, 43
meatloaf, 143
mint chocolate chip protein shake, 36
parmesan shrimp linguine, *144*, 145
shepherd's pie, 128
tomato basil omelette, *76*, 77
vanilla hazelnut protein shake, 37
vegetarian bolognese, 119

Oats
apple cinnamon oatmeal, 51
blueberry pie smoothie, 62
overnight oats, 72, *73*

pb & j overnight oats, 52
yogurt parfait, 50

Peanut Butter
apple peanut butter protein shake, 35
banana smoothie, 61
blueberry rice cake, 149, *154*, 155
chia seed pudding, 68
fruit dip, 153
overnight oats, 72, *73*
pb & j overnight oats, 52
protein bombs, 68, *69*
protein content, 19

Pork
stuffed pork chops, 116, *117*

Salads
apple pecan salad, 108, *109*
avocado feta & egg, 150, *151*
berry salad, 156
chicken grape & walnut, 94, *95*
chickpea tuna salad, 84, *85*
cobb salad, 82, *83*
greek salad, 152
roasted vegetable pasta salad, *130*, 131
taco salad, *102*, 103

Salmon
jalapeno cheddar salmon cakes, 98, *99*
one pan salmon and broccoli, 136
protein content, 19
sesame salmon wrap, 87

Soups
bean and vegetable soup, 97
broccoli cheddar soup, *56*, 57
butternut squash, 46
carrot ginger soup, 42
cauliflower asiago soup, 40, *41*
chicken tortilla, 100
cream of asparagus, 43
curry chickpea soup, *44*, 45
sausage and potato soup, 88, *89*
spring thyme vegetable soup, 53

sweet potato bisque, 47
vegetable chili, 54
white bean chili verde, 55

Spinach
bean and vegetable soup, 97
bean and walnut burgers, 92, *93*
cobb salad, 82, *83*
green smoothie, 60
loaded avocado toast, 70, *71*
meat & vegetable rice cake, 101
mediterranean frittata, 66, *67*
sausage and potato soup, 88, *89*
sesame salmon wrap, 87
stuffed bell peppers, 138, *139*
stuffed pork chops, 116, *117*
turkey & veg sandwich, 86

Sweet Potato
bisque, 47
black bean sweet potato tacos, 118
turkey tacos, 114, *115*
vegetable hash, 64, *65*

Taco
black bean sweet potato tacos, 118
salad, *102*, 103
turkey tacos, 114, *115*

Tuna
chickpea tuna salad, 84, *85*
dip, *154*, 155

Turkey
and veg sandwich, 86
and vegetable meatballs, 120, *121*
bacon swiss turkey burger, 140, *141*
cobb salad, 82, *83*
greek salad, 152
loaded avocado toast, 70, *71*
sausage chaffle, 75
turkey tacos, 114, *115*

Vegetarian
apple cinnamon oatmeal, 51

Vegetarian (cont'd)
apple pecan salad, 108, *109*
asparagus pesto chaffle, 104
bean and vegetable soup, 97
bean and walnut burgers, 92, *93*
black bean sweet potato tacos, 118
broccoli cheddar soup, *56*, 57
chia seed pudding, 68
chickpea burger with caesar salad, 96
fiesta cauliflower rice, 90, *91*
fruit smoothies, 58-62
garden vegetable chaffle, 101
grain-free granola, *78*, 79
liquid soups, 38-47
mashed cauliflower, 51
mediterranean frittata, 66, *67*
overnight oats, 72, *73*
pb & j overnight oats, 52
peanut butter protein bombs, 68, *69*
protein shakes, 30-37
roasted vegetable pasta salad, *130*, 131
southwest eggs, 50
spring thyme vegetable soup, 53
tomato basil omelette, 76, *77*
vegetable chili, 54
vegetarian bolognese, 119
yogurt parfait, 50

Yogurt
blueberry pie smoothie, 62
chicken & broccoli bake, 134, *135*
fruit dip, 153
grain-free granola, *78*, 79
green smoothie, 60
parfait, 50
parfait, 152
peanut butter banana smoothie, 61
pineapple mango smoothie, 61
protein content, 19
strawberry banana smoothie, 62
vegetable chili, 54
wild berry smoothie, 60

Made in the USA
Coppell, TX
18 November 2022